Rapid Review of

Clinical Medicine for MRCP Part 1

Rashmi Kaushal
BSc (Hons) MRCP (UK)
Consultant in Diabetes and Endocrinology
West Middlesex Hospital
Kingston, UK

Rikin Trivedi
BSc (Hons) MRCP (UK)
Research Fellow in Neurosciences
University of Cambridge
Cambridge, UK

Sanjay Sharma
BSc (Hons) MRCP (UK) MD
Consultant in Cardiology
University Hospital Lewisham
London, UK

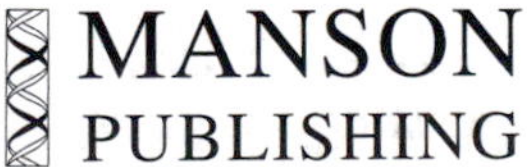

MANSON PUBLISHING

Dedication

For Ravi, Ashna, Anushka, Ishan, Asha, Shivani, Milan, and Priya.

ISBN: 1-84076-028-1

A CIP catalogue record for this book is available from the British Library.

For full details of all Manson Publishing Ltd titles please write to:
Manson Publishing Ltd, 73 Corringham Road, London NW11 7DL, UK.
Tel: +44(0)20 8905 5150
Fax: +44(0)20 8201 9233
Website: www.manson-publishing.com

Commissioning editor: Jill Northcott
Project manager: Paul Bennett
Copy-editor: Ruth Maxwell
Designer: Alpha Media
Cover photograph and design: Cathy Martin
Printed in India by Replika Press Pvt. Ltd.

Contents

Preface

Multiple-choice questions provide a standardized assessment of knowledge and continue to be the most popular method of examining medical students and doctors sitting postgraduate medical examinations. Conventionally, multiple-choice questions may use the 'true/false' format or the '1 from 5' format. The MRCP part 1 examination in the United Kingdom uses the latter format and consists of two papers, each containing 100 questions.

This book presents 350 '1 from 5' format questions similar in style and standard to those set by the Royal College of Physicians' examinations board and is aimed predominantly at doctors revising for the MRCP Part 1 examination. The book comprises 13 chapters dedicated to individual medical specialities: cardiology, respiratory medicine, haematology, renal medicine, neurology, rheumatology, gastroenterology, infectious diseases, endocrinology, psychiatry, dermatology, therapeutic medicine, and basic sciences. Detailed tutorials and revision lists are included in the answers that follow each question. The final (14th) chapter includes 100 questions from all of these specialities (in random order), which would normally constitute one paper in the MRCP Part 1 examination. The aim of this chapter is to provide the candidate with a mock examination to highlight individual strengths and weaknesses in knowledge and exam technique.

The book should also prove invaluable to senior medical students and doctors sitting other postgraduate examinations in internal medicine and PLAB examinations, and to lecturers in medicine. It is our aspiration that the knowledge derived from this book will provide a strong foundation for passing the MRCP part 1 and other similar postgraduate examinations.

Rashmi Kaushal
Rikin Trivedi
Sanjay Sharma

Acknowledgements

Our thanks are due to Dr Maria Androulika (Senior Clinical Fellow in Diabetes and Endocrinology) for her assistance with the Rheumatology chapter, Dr Parinaz Shams (Registrar in Ophthalmology) for assistance with the Neurology chapter, and to the first author's secretary, Valerie Symons for her tremendous support.

Finally, this book would not have been published in a timely fashion had it not been for the dedication and commitment of the editorial staff at Manson Publishing, with particular thanks to Paul Bennett, Ruth Maxwell, and Cathy Martin.

Abbreviations

AA (inflammatory) amyloid
ABPA allergic bronchopulmonary aspergillosis
ACE angiotensin converting enzyme
ACTH adrenocorticotrophic hormone
AD autosomal dominant
(L/R)AD axis deviation
ADH antidiuretic hormone
ADMA asymmetric dimethylarginine
AF atrial fibrillation
AIDS aquired immune deficiency syndrome
AIHA autoimmune haemolytic anaemia
ALL acute lymphoid leukaemia
ALP alkaline phosphatase
ALT alanine aminotransferase
AML acute myeloid leukaemia
ANCA anticytoplasmic antibody
ANF antinuclear factor
ANP atrial natriuretic peptide
APPT activated partial thromboplastin time
AR autosomal recessive
ARDS adult respiratory distress syndrome
ASD atrial septal defect
AST aspartate aminotransferase
ATN acute tubular necrosis
ATP adenosine triphosphate
AV atrio-ventricular
AVN atrio-ventricular node
AVNRT atrio-ventricular nodal re-entrant tachycardia
AVRT atrio-ventricular re-entrant tachycardia

(L/R)BBB (left/right) bundle branch block
BHL bilateral hilar lymphadenopathy
BOOP bronchiolitis obliterans organizing pneumonia
BP blood pressure
BSE bovine spongiform encephalopathy

CAH congenital adrenal hyperplasia
cAMP cyclic adenosine monophosphate
CAPD chronic ambulatory peritoneal dialysis
CBZ carbamazepine
CCF congestive cardiac failure
CEA carcinoembryonic antigen
CJD Creutzfeldt–Jakob disease
CK creatinine phosphokinase
CML chronic myeloid leukaemia
CMV cytomegalovirus
CNS central nervous system
CO carbon monoxide
COCP combined oestrogen contraceptive pill
COPD chronic obstructive pulmonary disease
COX cyclooxygenase
CRC chemokine receptor
CREST calcification Raynaud's esophageal telangiectasia
CRP C-reactive protein
CSF cerebrospinal fluid
CT computed tomography
CVA cerebral vascular accident
CXR chest X-ray

ddAVP desmopressin
DAF decay accelerating factor
DCT direct Coombs' test
DHEAS dehydroepiandrosterone sulphate
DI diabetes insipidus
DIC disseminated intravascular coagulation
DIG Digoxin Investigation Group
DIPJ distal interphalangeal joint
DKA diabetic ketoacidosis
DM diabetes mellitus
DMD Duchenne muscular dystrophy
DNA deoxyribonucleic acid
DPG diphosphoglycerate
DVT deep vein thrombosis

EBV Epstein–Barr virus
ECF extracellular fluid
ECG electrocardiogram
ECT electroconvulsive therapy
EDTA ethylene diamine tetra-acetic acid
EEG electroencephalogram
ELISA enzyme linked immuno-sorbant assay
EMG electromyogram
ENT ear, nose, and throat
ER endoplasmic reticulum
ERCP endoscopic retrograde cholangiopancreatography
ESR erythrocyte sedimentation rate

FP alpha fetoprotein
FAP familial adenomatous polyposis
FBC full blood count
FEV1 forced expiratory volume in first second
FSH follicle stimulating hormone
FTA fluorescent treponema antibodies
FVC forced vital capacity

G6PD glucose-6-phosphate dehydrogenase
GABA gamma aminobutyric acid
GBM glomerular basement membrane
GF growth factor
GF-r growth factor receptors
GFR glomerular filtration rate
GH growth hormone
GI gastrointestinal
GMP guanosine monophosphate
GN glomerulonephritis
GPI general paresis of insane
GSS Gerstmann–Straussler–Scheinker syndrome
GTP guanosine triphosphate

5-HIAA 5-hydroxyindole acetic acid
H&E haematoxylin and eosin stain
Hb haemoglobin
HbSC Sickle cell SC disease
HbSS Sickle cell disease
HCC hepatocellular carcinoma
HCG human chorionic gonadotrophin
HCM hypertrophic cardiomyopathy
HD haemodialysis
HepB sAg hepatitis B surface antigen
HHSV human herpes simplex virus
HIV human immunodeficiency virus
HLA human leukocyte antigen
HONC hyperosmolar nonketotic coma
HSP Henoch–Schonlein purpura
HSV herpes simplex virus
HT hypertension
HTLV human T-cell leukaemia virus

IBD irritable bowel disease
ICP intracranial pressure
IDDM insulin dependent diabetes

IFN interferon
Ig immunoglobulin
IGF insulin-like growth factor
IL interleukin
INO internucleur ophthalmoplegia
INR international normalized ratio
IQ intelligence quotient
ITP immune thrombocytopenia purpura
ITT insulin tolerance test
IV intravenous
IVC inferior vena cavae

JCA juvenile chronic arthritis
JVP jugular venous pulse/pressure

KCO transfer coefficient of carbon monoxide

LAP left atrial pressure
LDH lactate dehydrogenase
LDL low density lipoprotein
LFT liver function test
LMN lower motor neurone
L-NMMA N5-methyl L-arginine
LQTS long QT syndrome
LH luteinizing hormone
LMWH low molecular weight heparins
LUQ left upper quadrant
LVF left ventricular failure

MAC membrane attack complex
MAHA microangiopathic haemolytic anaemia
MAI *Mycobacterium avium intracellulariae*
MAO monoamine oxidase
MAOI monoamine oxidase inhibitor
MCH mean cell haemoglobin
MCP metacarpophalangeal
MCTD mixed connective tissue disease
MCV mean cell volume
MEN multiple endocrine neoplasia
MG myasthenia gravis
MI myocardial infarction
MPTP 1-methyl 4-phenyl 1,2,5,6-tetrahydropyridine
MR mitral regurgitation
MS multiple sclerosis
MVP mitral valve prolapse

NF neurofibromatosis
NIDDM noninsulin dependent diabetes mellitus
NK natural killer (cells)
NMJ neuromuscular junction
NO nitric oxide
NOS nitric oxide synthase
NSAID nonsteroidal anti-inflammatory drug
NYHA New York Heart Association

OA osteoarthritis
OCP oral contraceptive pill
OR odds ratio

PABA para-amino benzoic acid
PaO_2 partial pressure of oxygen in arterial blood
PAN polyarteritis nodosa
PAS periodic acid-Schiff
PBC primary biliary cirrhosis
PCO_2 partial pressure of carbon dioxide in arterial blood
PCP *Pneumocystis carinii*
PCR polymerase chain reaction
PCV packed cell volume
PDA patent ductus arteriosus
PE pulmonary embolus/i
PEFR peak expiratory flow rate
PG prostaglandin
PML progressive multifocal leucoencephalopathy
PMR polymyalgia rheumatica
PNH paroxysmal nocturnal haemoglobinuria
PPM permanent pacemaker
PPV positive predictive value
PR per rectum
PRP progressive rubella panencephalitis
PSA prostate specific antigen
PT prothrombin time
PTH parathyroid hormone
PTHrP parathormone related peptide
PTTK partial thromboplastin time
PUD peptic ulcer disease
PUO pyrexia of unknown origin

RA rheumatoid arthritis/right atrial
RAD right anterior descending
RBC red blood cell
RCT randomized controlled trial
RF rheumatoid factor
RFT respiratory function tests
RNA ribonucleic acid
RPGN rapidly proliferating glomerulonephritis
RTA renal tubular acidosis

SACD subacute combined degeneration of the cord
SAH subarachnoid haemorrhage
SAP serum amyloid protein
SD standard deviation
SDAT senile dementia of the Alzheimer's type
SEM standard error of the mean
SIADH syndrome of inappropriate antidiuretic hormone
SLE systemic lupus erythematosus
SOB shortness of breath
SSPE subacute sclerosing panencephalitis
STD sexually transmitted disease
SVC superior vena cavae
SVT supraventricular tachycardia

TB tuberculosis
TBG thyroid binding globulin
TCA tricarboxylic acid cycle/tricyclic antidepressant
TH T-helper (cell)
TIA transient ischaemic attack
TIBC total iron binding capacity
TLC total lung capacity
TLCO transfer factor
TNF tumour necrosis factor
TPHA *Treponema pallidum* haemagglutination assay
TPI *Treponema pallidum* immobilization
TPN total parenteral nutrition
TRBAb thyroid receptor blocking antibody
TRH thyroid releasing hormone
TSH thyroid stimulating hormone
TX treatment

UC ulcerative colitis
U+E urea & electrolytes
UMN upper motor neurone
UTI urinary tract infection

vWF von Willebrand's factor
VA alveolar volume
VDRL Venereal Disease Research Laboratory
(L/R)VEDP (left/right) ventricular end diastolic pressure
(L/R)VH (left/right) ventricular hypertrophy
VMA vanilyl mandellic acid
VQ ventilation/perfusion
VSD ventriculo-septal defect
VT ventricular tachycardia

WCC white cell count
WHO World Health Organization
WPW Wolff–Parkinson–White syndrome
WR Widal reaction

XR X-linked recessive

1 Applied Basic Sciences

Question 1 The following is not true for trinucleotide DNA repeats:

A Are highly polymorphic.
B Form a molecular explanation for genetic anticipation.
C Repeats coding for glutamine are neurotoxic.
D Are implicated in Friedreich's ataxia.
E Are stable during DNA replication.

Question 2 The following does not apply to the polymerase chain reaction:

A Is a technique that enables DNA amplification.
B Requires a DNA or RNA template.
C Uses oligonucleotide primers.
D Involves the freezing of nucleic acids.
E Is used in perinatal diagnosis.

Question 3 The following is true for xenotransplantation:

A The major target antigen is expressed in humans.
B Xenoreactive antibodies in the serum of the potential recipient form the basis of rejection.
C Rejection is acute.
D Genetic modification in the graft donor is contraindicated.
E T lymphocytes play a major role in rejection.

Question 4 The following is not true for cyclooxygenase:

A Is inhibited by NSAIDs.
B Acts on the substrate arachidonic acid.
C Are primarily involved in the synthesis of leukotrienes.
D COX1 is mainly associated with prostaglandin synthesis.
E Inhibition may lead to renal impairment.

Question 5 The following is true for prion disorders:

A May be inherited by an autosomal dominant trait.
B In the Gerstmann–Straussler–Scheinker syndrome the predominant disorder is a progressive dementia.
C CJD may manifest with ataxia.
D The incubation period is short.
E Transmission of nucleic acids is the infective agent.

Answer 1

E Are stable during DNA replication.

Trinucleotide repeats are a recent discovery which have provided a molecular explanation for the causes of a number of genetic neurological diseases. The repeats themselves consist of three nucleotides: CAG, CTG, CGG, and have been found in the coding and noncoding sequences of a number of genes. The number of repeats in the general population is variable as they are highly polymorphic.

The repeats are unstable during DNA replication and expansion may occur at this time. If this produces a long enough run of repeats, the gene is disrupted and the disease occurs. Repeats form the molecular explanation of genetic anticipation. Anticipation is the appearance of the disease at a progressively earlier age in successive generations and is caused by the expansion of the repeat element.

CTG codes for glutamine. This amino acid has been implicated in excitotoxic cell death in the CNS. It is believed that polyglutamine peptide sequences are themselves neurotoxic. Trinucleotide repeats have been implicated in:

- Fragile X syndrome.
- Huntington's disease.
- Friedreich's ataxia (and other hereditary ataxias).
- Myotonic dystrophy.
- Kennedy disease.

Answer 2

D Involves the freezing of nucleic acids.

The polymerase chain reaction is a technique that enables DNA amplification for the detection of specific gene sequences or markers.

First the region of interest in the DNA strand is located and 20–30 base pairs (oligonucleotides) at either end of this point are identified (and are known) as primers. These primers are mixed with a DNA template and a thermostable DNA polymerase. The DNA template is heated to enable it to unwind and hence form a single strand. As the template cools the primers will bind to the template of the appropriate sequence. The reaction is then heated to 72°C (140°F) and the DNA polymerase synthesizes new DNA between the two primer sequences. After 30+ cycles the target sequence will have been amplified exponentially and can be seen as a fluorescent band in an electrophoretic gel.

RNA can also be used as a template when it has been converted to complementary DNA (cDNA) by reverse transcriptase. In theory, it is possible to perform the technique using only one cell.

Uses of PCR include:

- Perinatal diagnosis for mutations.
- Single cell PCR can be performed on an *in vitro* fertilized embryo to confirm or exclude genetic abnormality prior to implantation.
- Detection of viral sequences, e.g. herpes virus in the CSF in suspected HSV encephalitis.

Answer 3

B Xenoreactive antibodies in the serum of the potential recipient form the basis of rejection.

Transplants performed between donor and recipient who belong to different species are known as xenotransplants or xenografts. The major target antigen is a galactose-containing disaccharide which is expressed in monkeys and pigs but not in humans. Rejection is caused by xenoreactive antibodies which are present in the serum of the potential human recipient. Rejection is hyperacute, occurring within hours or days post-transplant, and is characterized by rapid vascular spasm and occlusion resulting in failure of organ perfusion.

Genetic modification of donor complement control proteins DAF and CD59 may modify and reduce rejection. Studies have shown that enzymatic remodelling of the disaccharide antigen enables it to resemble human blood group molecules and hence serves to reduce rejection. T lymphocytes are not involved in the hyperacute rejection process.

Answer 4

C Are primarily involved in the synthesis of leukotrienes.

Cyclooxygenase is inhibited by all NSAIDs. Cyclooxygenase acts on arachidonic acid to form prostaglandins. Lipooxygenase acts on arachidonic acid to form leukotrienes. There are two isoforms of cyclooxygenase:

- COX1 is predominantly associated with the synthesis of prostaglandins which protect the gastric mucosa.
- COX2 is the inducible form which is involved in the inflammatory response.

Prostaglandins promote renal blood flow. Impaired production by NSAIDs can lead to renal impairment.

Tutorial

- PGE2, D2, F2alpha are involved in the inflammatory response.
- E2 is the most potent.
- They cause vasodilatation and potentiate the increase in permeability brought about by histamine and bradykinin.
- Prostaglandins also manifest anti-inflammatory effects by:
  - Suppressing release of polymorph lysosomal enzymes.
  - Reducing mast cell degranulation by raising intracellular cAMP levels.

Answer 5

A May be inherited by an autosomal dominant trait.

Prion particles are formed exclusively of protein, which is the infective agent. The do not contain nucleic acids. All cases of Gerstmann–Straussler–Scheinker syndrome (GSS) are of autosomal dominant (AD) inheritance with complete penetrance. Ten percent of all cases of CJD are also of AD inheritance. The mechanism underlying this is the transmission of the mutation prion protein gene.

In GSS the predominant clinical sign is ataxia which serves to distinguish it from CJD which manifests with a slowly progressive dementia and myoclonus. The incubation period is characteristically many years long. CJD is uncommon under the age of 50–65 years.

Histology shows extensive neuronal degeneration with astrocytic proliferation. There are also characteristic minute vesicles in the neurones and glial cells, resulting in the characteristic spongy change.

Other examples of prion disease include:

- Scrapie infection (sheep).
- Kuru (due to funeral practices).
- BSE.
- Fatal familial insomnia.

Question 6 The following is true for nitric oxide:

A Is formed from oxygen and nitrogen.
B Inhibits endothelial-derived relaxing factor.
C Synthesis may be activated by cytokines.
D Increases platelet aggregation.
E Reduces pulmonary blood flow.

Question 7 The following is not true for apoptosis:

A Is programmed cell death.
B Is associated with condensation of nuclear chromatin.
C Is inhibited by SLE.
D Occurs in graft-versus-host rejections.
E Is inhibited by methotrexate.

Answer 6

C Synthesis may be activated by cytokines.

Nitric oxide (NO) is synonymous with endothelium-derived relaxing factor.

It is a free radical gas and is generated from its substrate, L arginine, by the enzyme nitric oxide synthase (NOS).

$$\text{L Arginine} \xrightarrow[\text{NOS}]{} \text{Citruline} + \text{Nitric oxide}$$

Tutorial

There are at least three distinct forms of nitric oxide synthase:

- Inducible NOS (iNOS):
  - Found in macrophages.
  - Induced during cell-mediated immunity.
  - Activated by cytokines and antimicrobial products.
  - Plays a role in antimicrobial activity.
- Neuronal NOS (nNOS):
  - NO production is involved in regulation of neurotransmission.
  - Calcium/calmodulin dependent.
- Endothelial NOS:
  - NO production is involved in regulation of vascular tone.
  - Calcium/calmodulin dependent.
  - Activated by receptor G protein coupling in response to neurotransmitters, e.g. acetylcholine, substance P, and hormones, e.g. bradykinin.

Inhibition of NOS:
NOS is inhibited competitively by naturally occurring inhibitors which are found in the plasma such as:

- N5N5 dimethylarginine (asymmetrical dimethylarginine, ADMA).
- N5 methyl L arginine (L-NMMA).

Mechanism of action:
NO acts on target cells in close proximity to its site of synthesis. It activates guanylate cyclase leading to a rise in intracellular GMP which acts as a second messenger. It has a very short half-life.

Role of NO:

- NO is a vasodilator: in many tissues, vessels are maintained in tonic dilatation by NO. Infusion with a competitive inhibitor, e.g. L-NMMA, causes vasoconstriction.
- NO prevents platelet aggregation and adhesion to the vessel wall.
- NO favours cardiac filling during diastole: it increases cardiac compliance during diastole and reduces the duration of contraction. It has little effect on systolic contraction.
- NO may be antiatherogenic: it scavenges oxygen free radicals and prevents the attraction of inflammatory cells into the atheromatous lesions. Its activity is impaired by endothelial dysfunction leading to tonic vasoconstriction and vascular spasm. Its capacity to increase cyclic GMP will also have an antiproliferative effect.
- NO is a neurotransmitter both in the peripheral and central nervous systems (where it is thought to be important for memory formation).
- NO has been shown to be deficient in some cases of essential hypertension: studies on pre-eclamptic patients have also shown them to have much lower levels of NO when compared to pregnant normotensive controls. In septic shock, where there is abundant NO synthesis induced by cytokines and antimicrobial compounds, there is an associated hypotension.

Therapeutic effects of nitric oxide:

- NO is the active moiety in glyceryl trinitrate: it cannot, however, be infused as NO as it is unstable in solution resulting in the formation of toxic nitrites.
- NO can be therapeutically administered as a gas in a low concentration mixed with oxygen: the high avidity of Hb for NO enables rapid delivery following inhalation to the pulmonary vascular bed. It can be used in this manner to improve adult and neonatal respiratory distress. Inhaled NO also reverses pulmonary hypertension but its short half-life makes it difficult to use as a form of treatment.

Answer 7

E Is inhibited by methotrexate.

Apoptosis is programmed cell death. It is the mechanism underlying the elimination of single cells from living tissue. It is brought about by a stereotyped mechanism involving calcium- and magnesium-dependent endonucleases. In apoptosis the cell passes through the following stages:

- Condensation of chromatin in the nucleus.
- Deep invaginations of the nuclear membrane.
- Fragmentation of the nucleus.
- Contraction of the cytoplasm and aggregation of cytoplasmic organelles.
- Budding and separation of the membrane-bound bodies containing condensed organelles and nuclear fragments.

This converts the cell into several small apoptotic bodies which are usually phagocytosed by surrounding healthy tissue cells or by macrophages. If the intracellular contents are analyzed, a laboratory landmark of apoptosis is DNA laddering. Apoptosis does not provoke an acute inflammatory response.

SLE is associated with inhibition of apoptosis. Follicular lymphomas, breast and prostatic carcinoma, and oncogene bcl2 also inhibit cells from entering programmed cell death. Many chemotherapeutic agents, e.g. methotrexate, vincristine, cisplatin, doxarubicin induce apoptosis. Examples of apoptosis include:

- Loss of CD4 lymphocytes in HIV infection.
- Embryological development (more than 50% of motor neurones are removed).
- Certain viral infections affecting the liver (viral hepatitis, yellow fever).
- Cells dying as a result of T lymphocyte attack (chronic active hepatitis, graft-versus-host reactions).
- Clonal selection in the immune response.

Question 8 The following is not true for interferon:

A Are glycoproteins.
B IFN α has mainly antiviral actions.
C IFN γ activates macrophages.
D IFN α, β, and γ share the same receptor.
E Are effective in the treatment of HIV-related Kaposi's sarcoma.

Question 9 The following is not true for tumour necrosis factor:

A Is produced by the central necrotic core of cancers.
B Is the principal mediator of the host response to Gram-negative bacteria.
C Chronic overproduction causes cachexia.
D Acts as a pyrogen.
E Stimulates the release of stress hormones.

Answer 8

D IFN α, β, and γ share the same receptor.

Interferons are glycoprotein cytokines which help cells resist viral replication and regulate the immune response.

Tutorial

There are three types of interferons: α, β, γ:

IFNα and IFNβ:

- Are produced primarily by leucocytes and fibroblasts.
- Have mainly antiviral effects.
- Share a common receptor.
- The antiviral effects are mediated by the production of a protein kinase which phosphorylates the active site of the initiation factor responsible for protein synthesis and DNA replication in cells infected by the virus.

IFNγ:

- Is produced mainly by T lymphocytes and natural killer cells in response to antigenic (viral) stimulation.
- Activates macrophages.
- Promotes B-cell production of IgG.
- Interacts with a different receptor complex.

Therapeutic role of interferons:

IFNα is available in two forms (recombinant and lymphoblastoid).

Recombinant IFN α is used in the therapy of:

- Infection with hepatitis B and C in the chronic phase of disease.
- HIV-related Kaposi's sarcoma.
- Multiple myeloma.
- Advanced non-Hodgkin's lymphoma.

Lymphoblastoid IFNα is mainly used in the treatment of hairy cell leukaemia.

Side-effects of treatment with interferons include:

- Myelosuppression.
- Hypotension.
- Cardiac arrhythmias.
- Pulmonary infiltrates.

Answer 9

A Is produced by the central necrotic core of cancers.

Tumour necrosis factor (TNF) derives its name from the fact that it kills tumour cells directly in culture. This is unlikely to be the case *in vivo*. There are two types of TNF (α and β). TNFα is now regarded as the central mediator of the pathophysiological changes that occur in the host following the release of lipopolysaccharide from bacterial cell walls.

Tutorial

TNFα:

- Has many features in common with IL-1.
- Is synthesized by macrophages, T lymphocytes, natural killer cells, and Kuppfer cells in response to infection and inflammation.
- Its effects depend on its concentration and duration of production. In small amounts it has beneficial effects on inflammation and tissue repair, whereas sudden systemic release may result in shock and tissue injury.
- Chronic overproduction results in cachexia.

Role of TNFα in inflammation:

- Enhances chemotaxis of macrophages and polymorphs.
- Increases phagocytosis and cytotoxic activity.

Role of TNFα as a pyrogen:

- By direct effect on the hypothalamus.
- By inducing IL-1 synthesis.

Role of TNFα in tissue repair:

- It has an important role in tissue remodelling due to its proliferative and destructive properties.
- It can stimulate proliferation of fibroblasts and endothelial cells, and induces synthesis of growth factors.
- On the other hand, it can be directly cytotoxic to endothelial cells and promotes the synthesis of proteases active against the connective tissue matrix.

Role of TNFα in septic shock:
It is the central mediator in septic shock complicating conditions such as Gram-negative septicaemia. Its effects include:

- Fever.
- Respiratory arrest.
- Lactic acidosis.
- The release of stress hormones.

Role of TNFα in cachexia:
Long term overproduction results in:

- Anorexia with loss of fat and protein.
- Anaemia.
- Increased acute phase protein synthesis.
- Hypertriglyceridaemia.

TNFβ:
TNFβ is also known as lymphotoxin. It has similar effects as TNFα and is also responsible for lymphocyte-mediated tissue destruction.

Question 10 The following is not true for protooncogenes:

A Are found in viral cells.
B May code for growth factors.
C May act by receptor amplification.
D Point mutations in the GTPase-binding proteins are involved in the pathogenesis of colorectal carcinoma.
E Activation may result from translocation.

Question 11 The following is not true for the structure of immunoglobulin:

A Consists of two heavy chains and two light chains linked by disulphide bonds.
B The Fc fragment is able to bind to antigens.
C The light chains may be of the kappa (κ) or lambda (λ) type.
D Half of each light chain and a quarter of each heavy chain has a variable (v) region.
E The joining of v regions to joining (j) regions is imprecise and adds to diversity of antibody structure.

Question 12 The following is true for immunoglobulin IgE:

A Present in the normal serum in a concentration similar to that of IgG.
B Are attached to macrophages in the skin.
C Involved in type II hypersensitivity mechanisms.
D Transmitted across the normal placenta.
E Found in a high concentration in the serum of patients with atopic eczema.

Answer 10

A Are found in viral cells.

Oncogenes are genes either viral or mammalian in origin that cause transformation of cells in culture. In normal cells, they are switched off or down regulated. Copies in viral cells are known as V-oncogenes, while in mammalian cells they are known as c-onc or protooncogenes.

Tutorial

Protooncogenes fall into four groups:

Growth factors (GF):
- Increased or inappropriate production of growth factors.
- Loss of production of inhibitory growth factors.

Growth factor receptors (GF-r):
- Increased number of receptors by overexpression or amplification of the GF-r gene, e.g. *erb-B*, *erb-B2* gene in breast cancer.
- Abnormal receptors which do not require GF stimulation.

Signal transduction:
- Point mutations in GTPase-binding proteins increasing the level of signal transmission, e.g. ras family in colorectal carcinoma; gsp in pituitary adenoma.
- Overexpression of GTPase proteins or tyrosine kinases increasing the level of signal transduction.
- Translocation of tyrosine kinase to form a new protein product with increased activity, e.g. abl-bcr in chronic myeloid leukaemia.

Nuclear factors:
- Gene amplification of cell cycle control proteins, e.g. n-myc in neuroblastoma.

No protooncogenes involved in the synthesis of complement proteins have been described.

Oncogene activation:
Oncogenes may be activated by a variety of methods. These include:
- Point mutations resulting in increased signal transmission.
- Amplification resulting in increased numbers of genes increasing protein synthesis.
- Translocation and gene fusion resulting in the formation of a new protein.
- Insertion of viral genome resulting in increased transcription of a gene.

Answer 11

B The Fc fragment is able to bind to antigens.

Immunoglobulins share a similar basic structure, and consist of two heavy and two light polypeptide chains linked by disulphide bonds. The Fab fragment is capable of binding antigens, the Fc fragment is not. Light chains are of two types, kappa (κ) and lambda (λ), and each immunoglobulin molecule has either 2κ or 2λ chains but never one of each.

The heavy chains are of five types (γ, α, μ, δ, ε) and each molecule has the same type. Five distinct immunoglobulins are recognized on the basis of their heavy chains: IgG, IgA, IgM, IgD, and IgE. Half of each light chain and a quarter of each heavy chain consists of a variable (v) region.

The initial germ line DNA contains genes which code for different variable and constant (c) regions, as well as genes which code for the amino acids of the joining region (j), joining c and v segments. The joining of v to j regions is imprecise, adding further diversity to antibody structure. Further diversity is introduced in the production of heavy chains.

Answer 12

E Found in a high concentration in the serum of patients with atopic eczema.

IgE is only present in trace amounts in the immunological pool and has a molecular weight of 190,000 daltons. It has a special property of being able to attach to tissue, particularly to mast cells and basophils, by means of its Fc fragment, leaving the specific combining sites on the Fab fragments available for union with antigen.

IgE is involved in type I hypersensitivity reactions which occur in conditions such as atopic asthma or eczema. When attached to mast cells, exposure to an allergen triggers the mast cell to degranulate and release mediators, producing the type I reaction. It is IgG and IgM that are involved in the cytotoxic type II hypersensitivity reactions.

IgE may play a role in helminthic reactions.

Tutorial

IgG:
- Is the major serum immunoglobulin accounting for 70% of the immunological pool.
- Molecular weight 150,000 daltons.
- Properties:
  - Crosses the placental barrier and is therefore the major protective immunoglobulin to the neonate.
  - Diffuses easily into all extracellular fluids.
  - Acts as an antitoxin (neutralizing antibody).
  - Responsible for opsonic binding of bacteria.
  - Complement activation by two or more molecules through their Fc portion.

IgA:
- Represents 15–20% of the immunological pool.
- Molecular weight 160,000+ daltons.
- Properties:
  - Is the principal immunoglobulin found in secretions such as breast milk, saliva, tears, sweat, and GI secretions.
  - Prevents infection of mucous membranes by inhibiting adhesion of organisms to the epithelium.
  - When aggregated will bind polymorphs and activate complement by the alternative pathway.

IgM:
- Represents 10% of the immunological pool.
- Molecular weight 900,000 daltons.
- Properties:
  - Produced early in response to infection.
  - Largely restricted to plasma.
  - Acts as an agglutinating and opsonizing antibody.

Question 13 The following is true for atrial natriuretic peptide:

A Consists of 124 amino acids.
B Causes hypertension.
C Levels are reduced in the presence of an expanded extracellular volume.
D Promotes renal loss of sodium.
E Receptors are present in the kidney.

Question 14 The following is true for changes occuring during pregnancy:

A Increase in serum creatinine.
B Reduction in red cell mass.
C An increase in the basal metabolic rate.
D An increase in renal blood flow by 50%.
E A reduction in total serum thyroxine.

Question 15 The following is true for the actions of insulin:

A Promotes lipolysis in adipose tissue.
B Inhibits glucose uptake by muscle.
C Inhibits gluconeogenesis in the liver.
D Actions are potentiated by oestrogens.
E Actions are reinforced by growth hormone.

Answer 13

D Promotes renal loss of sodium.

Atrial natriuretic peptide (ANP) is a 28-amino acid polypeptide. It is secreted by the atria in response to stretching of the atrial myocardium. Expansion of the ECF, e.g. in congestive cardiac failure, is associated with stretching of the atria and release of ANP.

ANP promotes renal loss of water and sodium and hence causes hypotension. Other actions include a reduction in vascular smooth muscle responsiveness to vasoconstrictor substances and inhibition of the secretion of aldosterone.

Answer 14

C An increase in the basal metabolic rate.

The serum urea and creatinine are reduced during pregnancy due to increased clearance by the kidney. There is an increase in the red cell mass and plasma volume. The basal metabolic rate is increased with a resultant increase in oxygen consumption by 25%. Renal blood flow is also increased by 25% while the GFR is increased by 50%. Other changes include an increase in cardiac output, heart rate, and stroke volume. In the blood there is a reduction in serum iron and Hb with an associated increase in transferrin and TIBC.

During pregnancy, there is a significant increase in the thyroid binding globulin and hence an increase in the total plasma thyroxine levels. Other causes of an increase in thyroid binding globulin include oral contraceptives and oestrogen therapy, hypothyroidism, drugs such as phenothiazines, and viral infections, particularly acute viral hepatitis.

Similarly, thyroid binding globulin may be reduced in thyrotoxicosis, androgen treatment, Cushing's syndrome, nephrotic syndrome, and any major illness or malnutrition.

Answer 15

C Inhibits gluconeogenesis in the liver.

Insulin is an anabolic hormone. In adipose tissue, insulin increases fatty acid synthesis and storage, and inhibits lipolysis. It increases glucose uptake in adipose tissue and muscle, and in the liver where it promotes glycogen synthesis and lipogenesis. It inhibits gluconeogenesis and ketogenesis.

In the muscle, insulin increases amino acid uptake with increased protein and glycogen synthesis. The actions of insulin are antagonized by oestrogens, growth hormone, thyroxine, glucagon, and cortisol.

2 Cardiology

Question 1 Right bundle branch block is a characteristic finding in:

A 10% of the healthy general population.
B Atrial septal defect.
C Left ventricular hypertrophy.
D Hypertrophic cardiomyopathy.
E Coarctation of the aorta.

Question 2 The following is true on the 12-lead ECG:

A The QT interval in a patient with a heart rate of 60 beats per minute is >440 msec.
B A PR interval exceeding 200 msec is normal in sinus bradycardia.
C The P-wave in lead V1 exceeding 0.25mV is suggestive of left atrial hypertrophy.
D The sum of the R-wave in V1 and the S-wave in V6 should not exceed 2 mV.
E T-wave inversion exceeding 0.3 mV in the limb leads is always abnormal.

Question 3 Congenital long QT syndrome:

A Is a common cause of sudden death in young adults.
B Is due to abnormalities in sodium or potassium ion channels in the myocardium.
C Is best treated with isoprenaline.
D Right stellate ganglionectomy is a recognized form of therapy.
E May be due to a mutation in the gene encoding the sarcomeric contractile protein troponin.

Question 4 The following is a recognized ECG change of hypokalaemia:

A Short PR interval.
B Tall T-waves.
C J-waves.
D Widening of the QRS complex.
E ST segment elevation.

Answer 1

B Atrial septal defect.

Right bundle branch block is characterized by a broad QRS complex with a dominant R-wave in V1. The characteristic complex is characterized by a rsR pattern. In addition, there is a prominent S-wave in V6. It is found in 1% of the healthy general population and is a recognized finding in any case of right ventricular hypertrophy or overload, for example ASD, VSD, Fallot's, pulmonary stenosis, pulmonary emboli, and cor pulmonale (smoking, lung fibrosis, chronic lung suppuration). Other causes of RBBB include:

- Acute myocardial infarction, particularly anterior infarction.
- Cardiomyopathies (which may also cause LBBB).
- Conduction tissue disease (which may also cause LBBB).
- Right ventriculotomy.
- Hyperkalaemia.
- Class 1a antiarrhythymic agents.

Coarctation of the aorta and hypertension are characteristically associated with voltage criteria of left ventricular hypertrophy. Whilst almost any ECG abnormality is possible in hypertrophic cardiomyopathy, most patients exhibit deep S waves in the septal leads and/or pathological q waves in the inferior or lateral leads.

Answer 2

E T-wave inversion exceeding 0.3 mV in the limb leads is always abnormal.

The normal corrected QT interval should not exceed 440 msec. The formula for correcting the QT for the heart rate is QT measured in seconds/square root of the RR interval in seconds. At a heart rate of 60 the RR interval in seconds is 1. The square root of 1 is also 1, therefore the corrected QT of <440 msec (0.44 sec) is normal. A QT (corrected for heart rate) exceeding 440 msec is prolonged.

Causes of long QT
Inherited disorders:

- Romano–Ward (autosomal dominant) and Jarvell–Lange–Neilsen (autosomal recessive which is also associated with sensorineuronal deafness).

Drugs:

- Class 1a and 1c and class III antiarrhythmic agents.
- Neuroleptic agents.
- Tricyclic antidepressants.
- Antihistamines such as terfenadine and astemizole.
- Erythromycin.

Electrolyte disturbances:

- Hyokalaemia, hypocalcaemia, hypomagnesaemia.

Organophosphate poisoning.

Cardiac causes:

- Sick sinus syndrome.
- Complete heart block.
- Bradycardia.
- Mitral valve prolapse.
- Myocardial infarction.

Miscellaneous:

- Subarachnoid haemorrhage.

Right atrial enlargement is characterized by a large P-wave exceeding 0.25 mV in both II and V1. Left atrial enlargement is characterized by a P-wave exceeding 0.12 seconds in duration in II (bifid shape), and a biphasic P-wave in lead V1 where the terminal portion is more than 0.1 mV and 0.04 secs in duration (in other words more than 1 small square deep and more than 1 small square wide).

Sinus bradycardia does not result in a prolonged PR interval although certain anti-arrhythmic drugs, hyperkalaemia, and regular intensive physical training may cause both.

The Sokolow voltage criteria for RVH is the R-wave in V1 plus S-wave in V6 exceeding 1.25 mV. The Sokolow voltage criteria for LVH is the S-wave in V1 plus the R-wave in V6 exceeding 3.5 mV. T-wave inversion exceeding –0.3 mV is always pathological.

Answer 3

B Is due to abnormalities in sodium or potassium ion channels in the myocardium.

Congenital long QT syndrome (LQTS) is a recognized but rare cause of sudden death in young adults. Death is due to polymorphic tachycardia (torsades de points) degenerating into ventricular fibrillation. Syncope is common in affected patients and is due to transient cerebral hypoperfusion from ventricular tachycardia. Common stimuli for polymorphic VT include physical exertion, intense emotion, and auditory stimuli.

Genes encoding sodium and potassium ion channels cause disease. To date there are seven different loci on chromosomes 3, 4, 7, and 11. On chromosome 7 there is a mutation in the HERG gene (potassium channel abnormality). Other mutations include the SCN5A (chromosome 3: sodium ion channels) and KVLQT1 (chromosome 11: potassium ion channels). It has been postulated that there is an imbalance of sympathetic drive between the left and right stellate side.

Management involves beta-blockers in the first instance. If this is unsuccessful then a left stellate ganglionectomy is carried out. Implantable cardiovertor defibrillators are being increasingly employed in the management of congenital LQTS patients with recurrent syncopal episodes. Isoprenaline, a sympathomimetic agent, is contraindicated in the treatment of congenital LQTS, although it has an important place in the management of acquired LQTS where the aim is to keep the heart rate above 60 bpm (isoprenaline or atrial pacing) until the underlying cause has been treated. Mutations within genes encoding sarcomeric contractile proteins such as troponin cause hypertophic and dilated cardiomyopathy.

Answer 4

D Widening of the QRS complex.

Hypokalaemia is characterized by:
- Flattening of the T-waves.
- Prominent U-waves.
- Increased PR interval.
- Increased QT interval.
- Widening of the QRS complexes.
- ST segment depression.

J-waves are a feature of hypothermia although they may also occur in normothermic patients. U-waves are not specific to hypokalaemia and may be seen in LVH and bradycardia and in patients on digoxin. There is good correlation between serum potassium levels <3 mmol/l and ECG changes.

ST segment elevation occurs in myocardial infarction, coronary artery spasm, and pericarditis.

A short PR interval is a feature of pre-excitation syndromes but also may occur in sinus tachycardia, AV nodal re-entrant tachycardias, hypertrophic cardiomyopathy, Pompe's disease, and Duchenne muscular dystrophy.

Question 5 The following statement is true of hypertrophic cardiomyopathy:

A Over 60% of cases are familial.
B The prevalence is 0.001%.
C Hypertrophic cardiomyopathy is the commonest cause of sudden cardiac death in athletes aged over 25 years.
D Concentric left ventricular hypertrophy is the commonest pattern of hypertrophy.
E The vast majority of patients have resting left ventricular outflow obstruction.

Question 6 In hypertrophic cardiomyopathy:

A A left ventricular outflow tract murmur is invariably present.
B The carotid pulse is slow rising.
C Auscultation of the precordium often reveals a third heart sound.
D Systolic function is impaired in the majority of patients.
E The apex is often displaced.

Question 7 The murmur across the left ventricular outflow tract in hypertrophic cardiomyopathy:

A Varies with posture.
B Is decreased by dehydration.
C Is not affected by nitrates.
D Is reduced by digoxin.
E Is increased by passive leg raising.

Answer 5

A Over 60% of cases are familial.

Hypertrophic cardiomyopathy is a very common exam topic. It is defined as ventricular hypertrophy in the absence of a cardiac or systemic cause. The condition is familial in over 70% of cases with autosomal dominant inheritance. The prevalence is 0.1–0.2%. Sudden death is well recognized. The annual mortality is 2.5–6% per annum. HCM is the commonest cause of sudden cardiac death in young athletes. Asymmetrical septal hypertrophy is the commonest pattern of hypertrophy, occurring in 60% of cases. Thirty percent of patients have concentric hypertrophy and 10% have hypertrophy confined to the apex. Mutations within genes encoding sarcomeric contractile proteins cause disease. The condition is genetically heterogeneous and to date there are abnormalities within genes on four chromosomal loci (See Table). Resting left ventricular outflow obstruction is present in around 25% of patients.

Chromosome	*Gene affected*
14	β myosin heavy chain
1	troponin T
15	α tropomyosin
11	myosin-binding protein C

Answer 6

E The apex is often displaced.

In hypertrophic cardiomyopathy a left ventricular outflow tract murmur is present in just 25% of patients at rest. This is due to a combination of asymmetrical septal hypertrophy and systolic anterior motion of the mitral valve apparatus. The carotid pulse is 'jerky' in patients with obstruction. A slow rising pulse occurs in aortic stenosis. A fourth heart sound is common due to forceful atrial contraction against a stiff ventricle. A third heart sound is unusual because ventricular relaxation is impaired and ventricular filling is relatively slow (Note: third heart sound occurs with rapid ventricular filling).

The apex is often displaced in hypertrophic cardiomyopathy due to the severe left ventricular hypertrophy. Ninety percent of patients have hyperdynamic systolic function. Symptoms of heart failure are due to diastolic dysfunction. The other 10% develop progressive dilatation of the left ventricle usually in middle age and usually have a poor prognosis.

Answer 7

A Varies with posture.

The left ventricular outflow obstruction is increased in conditions causing reduced left ventricular end diastolic pressure, either by reducing preload or afterload. This results in an increase in the intensity of the outflow tract murmur heard in obstructive HCM. Standing suddenly causes a transient increase in obstruction due to reduced preload. Conversely, squatting, repeated hand grip, or passive leg raising increases preload by facilitating blood flow to the heart. Fluid loss from any source, vasodilatation, and inotropes will also reduce left ventricular end diastolic pressure (see Tutorial).

Tutorial

Factors increasing and decreasing outflow tract obstruction:

	Contractility	*Preload*	*Afterload*
Increased obstruction			
Valsalva manoeuvre	—	↓	↓
Standing suddenly	—	↓	—
Hypovolaemia	↑	↓	↓
Digitalis	↑	↓	↓
Vasodilators	—	↓	↓
Decreased obstruction			
Squatting	—	↑	↑
Passive leg raising	—	↑	↑
Beta-blockers	↓	↑	—

Question 8 The following is true of mitral valve prolapse:

A Is commoner in males than females.
B Is associated with hypothyroidism.
C Syncopal episodes are recognized.
D Increases the risk of infective endocarditis in all affected patients.
E Is a common cause of sudden cardiac death.

Question 9 In the management of myocardial infarction the following is an absolute contraindication to thrombolysis:

A Menstruation.
B Left bundle branch block.
C Absent carotid pulse and an early diastolic murmur in a patient presenting with myocardial infarction.
D Previous myocardial infection.
E Systolic blood pressure <100 mmHg (13.3 kPa).

Question 10 The following patients have the greatest benefit when treated with thrombolysis:

A Posterior myocardial infarction.
B Patients treated within the first 36 hours of onset of chest pain.
C Patients with ST segment depression in the anterior leads.
D Patients with inferior myocardial infarction.
E Patients presenting with new BBB and chest pain consistent with myocardial infarction.

Question 11 In a patient with a broad complex tachycardia, which of the following favours ventricular tachycardia:

A P waves following each QRS complex.
B Heart rate of 120/minute.
C Termination with adenosine.
D Dissociated P-waves.
E Reduced heart rate with carotid sinus massage.

Answer 8

C Syncopal episodes are recognized.

Mitral valve prolapse (MVP) is common in the general population. True MVP is present in approximately 5%. The incidence is higher in females. It is the commonest cardiac manifestation of Marfan's syndrome. Other associations include hypertrophic cardiomyopathy, thyrotoxicosis, ASD, WPW syndrome, and LQTS. Hypothyroidism is not associated with the condition. The condition is generally benign.

Symptoms include atypical chest pain which is sharp in nature and localized in the inframammary region, breathlessness on exertion even in the presence of normal cardiac function, transient dizziness, and syncope. On examination there may be a single or multiple systolic clicks or a high pitched midsystolic murmur. Approximately 10% of patients go on to develop significant mitral regurgitation (MR).

MVP increases the risk of endocarditis and antibiotic prophylaxis before dental or invasive genitourinary/lower bowel procedures is recommended in patients *who have MR only*. In the absence of MR prophylaxis is not necessary. Transient ischaemic attacks occur in a very small proportion of patients and sudden death in association with MVP is recognized. However, whether the post mortem findings are causal or coincidental is debatable. It is possible that the very small number of patients who have died suddenly had associated LQTS or WPW.

Answer 9

C Absent carotid pulse and an early diastolic murmur in a patient presenting with myocardial infarction.

Thrombolysis has revolutionized the management of myocardial infarction. It has been widely used since the early 1980s. Thrombolytic therapy is associated with an 18% improvement in mortality (23 lives saved per 1000 patients treated). The contraindications are as follows:

Absolute:
- Suspected aortic dissection.
- Active bleeding (includes retinal bleed in diabetics).
- Previous cerebral haemorrhage.
- Cerebral neoplasm.

Major:
- Major surgery within 2 weeks.
- Head injury or thrombotic/embolic CVA within 2 months.
- Severe gastrointestinal bleeding within 2 weeks.
- Heavy vaginal bleeding.

Minor:
- Previous history of thrombotic or embolic CVA.
- Use of anticoagulants.
- Pregnancy.
- Suspected allergic reaction.
- Uncontrolled systolic blood pressure >180 mmHg (24 kPa).
- Active peptic ulcer disease, chronic liver disease, pancreatitis.
- Diabetic retinal neovascularization.

Pregnancy is *not* an absolute contraindication. Hypotension is also not an absolute contraindication for thrombolysis. Indeed it may be suggestive of cardiogenic shock in which early coronary patency may be life saving. However, streptokinase should be avoided in hypotensive patients as the drug itself may lower blood pressure in some patients. Streptokinase (but not other thrombolytic agents) should also be avoided in patients who may have received the drug during previous myocardial infarction. A patient with myocardial infarction, absent carotid pulse, and aortic regurgitation should raise the suspicion of aortic dissection and should not be thrombolyzed until dissection has been confidently excluded. Patients with myocardial infarction who present with LBBB receive great benefit from thrombolysis.

Answer 10

E Patients presenting with LBBB and chest pain consistent with myocardial infarction.

All patients with ST segment elevation of 2 mm or more in contiguous chest leads or 1 mm or more in contiguous limb leads benefit from thrombolysis, provided therapy is initiated within 12 hours (ideally 4 hours). Patients with anterior myocardial infarction benefit most compared with infarction affecting the inferior or lateral wall. Patients with posterior infarcts classically present with ST segment depression. In posterior myocardial infarction, patients classically have deep ST segment depression in the anterior leads. Thrombolysis in patients with ST segment depression has been associated with increased mortality primarily due to the potential haemorrhagic complications.

Elderly patients have derived the greatest benefit from thrombolysis since mortality prior to the thrombolytic era was much higher in patients above the seventh decade. Patients with acute myocardial infarction presenting with LBBB have a high mortality without thrombolysis, and according to pooled data thrombolysis saves 25 lives per 1000 treated. The greatest benefit from thrombolysis occurs in:
- Anterior MI.
- MI/LBBB.
- Older patients.
- Patients treated within 4 hours of onset of symptoms.

Answer 11

D Dissociated P-waves.

The differential diagnosis of a broad complex tachycardia is between ventricular tachycardia, nodal tachycardia, and supraventricular tachycardia with aberrant conduction. The difficulty is differentiating some cases of VT from the SVT plus aberrant conduction. The ventricular rate is similar in both. Ventricular tachycardia should be suggested by the following:

- Extreme axis deviation.
- rsR pattern in V1 (rabbit's left ear if he was looking at you!).
- Concordance in all the chest leads, i.e. all QRS complexes (except V1 which is usually positive) negative or positive.
- Fusion and capture beats.
- Dissociated P-waves.

In addition, a history of ischaemic heart disease lends further support to the diagnosis of VT, as does the presence of Cannon waves (AV dissociation) on the JVP. Carotid sinus massage has no effect on heart rate in VT, whereas it may transiently slow or terminate SVT. Adenosine is characteristically useful in the terminating SVT and should help differentiate between SVT and VT. However, VT arising from the right ventricular outflow tract may also respond to adenosine.

Question 12 In a patient with a broad complex tachycardia, which of the following favours supraventricular tachycardia:

A Regular P-waves buried in the QRS complex.
B Extreme left axis deviation.
C Upright QRS complexes in all chest leads.
D Fusion beats.
E Onset due to ventricular ectopic on the preceding T-wave.

Question 13 A third heart sound:

A Is due to forced atrial contraction against a stiff ventricle.
B Is common in aortic stenosis.
C Is a recognized finding in mitral stenosis.
D Is an uncharacteristic finding in young athletes.
E Occurs in pericardial constriction.

Question 14 The following are cardiac catheter data on a 26-year-old female with a murmur:

Chamber pressure	*mmHg (kPa)*	*Oxygen saturation (%)*
SVC		66
IVC		63
Upper right atrium	9 (1.2)	66
Mid right atrium	12 (1.6)	92
Lower right atrium	12 (1.6)	92
Right ventricle	40/9 (5.3/1.2)	92
Pulmonary artery	40/15 (5.3/2.0)	92
Left ventricle	110/3 (14.7/0.4)	99
Pulmonary capillary wedge	6 (0.8)	

Which of the following statements is true?

A The patient is likely to be clubbed.
B A right ventricular heave is highly likely to be present on examination.
C There will be a harsh pansystolic at the left lower sternal edge.
D The ECG will demonstrate left axis deviation and RBBB.
E The second heart sound will be soft.

Answer 12

A Regular P-waves buried in the QRS complex.

In SVT with aberrant conduction, the P-waves may be visible buried within the QRS complex or occur just after the QRS complex (AVNRT) in a regular fashion. In VT P-waves may also be seen buried with QRS complexes; however, these are very irregular. The rhythm disturbance is often preceeded by an atrial ectopic beat. VT may be initiated by R on T phenomenon where a ventricular ectopic falls on the preceeding R-wave. Carotid sinus massage or other vagotonic manoeuvres slow down the heart rate in SVT and often terminate the arrhythmia. In contrast the heart rate in VT is unaffected by such measures. The presence of a slurred R-wave in sinus rhythm (delta wave) is very suggestive of WPW syndrome which is associated with SVT rather than VT. Extreme axis deviation (left or right) is more characteristic of VT.

Answer 13

E Occurs in pericardial constriction.

The third heart sound is due to rapid filling of either ventricle. It is a low pitched sound occurring shortly after the second heart sound and is best heard with the bell of the stethoscope. A third heart sound is common in children and in fit subjects. It is also heard during a tachycardia in some healthy individuals. In older subjects (fifth decade) a third heart sound is usually pathological and most commonly due to systolic ventricular dysfunction. Other pathological causes of a third heart sound include mitral regurgitation, aortic regurgitation, pericardial constriction, cardiac tamponade, and restrictive cardiomyopathy. A third heart sound is never heard in conditions where rapid flow into the ventricles during diastole is prevented, such as mitral stenosis or tricuspid stenosis. In pericardial constriction the sudden rush of blood into the ventricles during diastole causes a very loud third heart sound which is often termed the 'pericardial knock'.

A fourth heart sound is due to forced atrial contraction against a stiff ventricle and it may also be normal in highly trained athletes and children. Pathological causes of a fourth heart sound include ventricular dysfunction (left or right), hypertrophic cardiomyopathy, aortic stenosis, hypertension, and coarctation of the aorta.

Answer 14

B A right ventricular heave is highly likely to be present on examination.

There is increased right atrial pressure, right ventricular pressure and pulmonary artery pressure. There is also a step up in oxygen saturation at the level of the right atrium (midportion) suggesting an ostium secundum atrial septal defect with a left to right shunt. The patient will not be cyanosed. There may be a palpable right ventricular heave given the elevated right heart pressures. A middiastolic murmur may be heard in the tricuspid area due to the increased flow across the tricuspid valve in diastole. An ejection systolic flow murmur in the pulmonary area is more characteristic of ASD, as is fixed splitting of the second heart sound.

The ECG would, in an ostium secundum ASD, usually demonstrate right axis deviation and partial RBBB. In addition, there may be deep S-waves in V5 and V6 when right ventricular hypertrophy is present. In contrast, the ECG in ostium primum ASD reveals left axis deviation and partial RBBB +/– RVH. In addition there may be ECG evidence of left atrial hypertrophy due to associated mitral regurgitation due to a cleft anterior mitral valve leaflet.

Question 15 The jugular venous pressure:

A Is elevated in gastrointestinal haemorrhage.
B Is reduced during deep inspiration.
C May demonstrate large v-waves in tricuspid stenosis.
D Prominent a-waves are a recognized feature of tricuspid regurgitation.
E Rises during expiration in pericardial constriction.

Question 16 Cannon waves are present in:

A Atrial fibrillation.
B Supraventricular tachycardia.
C Electromechanical dissociation.
D Multiple ventricular ectopics.
E Mobitz 2 AV block.

Question 17 Ostium secundum ASD:

A Account for more than 50% of all ASDs.
B A long PR interval on the ECG is a common finding.
C LBBB on the ECG is well recognized.
D Is associated with ventricular arrhythmias.
E Affected patients often have an absent spleen.

Question 18 The following is true for WPW syndrome:

A Narrow QRS complex.
B Slurred R-wave.
C Is always familial.
D Digoxin is the drug of choice in atrial fibrillation secondary to WPW syndrome.
E Verapamil is the drug of choice in supraventricular tachycardia secondary to WPW syndrome.

Answer 15

B Is reduced during deep inspiration.

The JVP is a measure of the right atrial pressure. The absence of valves in the internal jugular vein allows transmission of right atrial pressure directly to the neck veins. The JVP is increased in conditions which elevate right atrial pressure. These include volume overload (acute renal failure), congestive cardiac failure, tricuspid stenosis or regurgitation, pulmonary stenosis, pulmonary hypertension, pericardial constriction, and cardiac tamponade. The central venous pressure is reduced by deep inspiration; however, in pericardial constriction there is a paradoxical increase (Kussmaul's sign). The normal wave form consists of:

- a-wave: due to atrial contraction.
- c-wave: due to ventricular systole (tricuspid valve is pushed upwards slightly during systole).
- v-wave: which results from passive filling of the atrium.

The a-wave is followed by an x descent (tricuspid valve pulled down just before systole) and the v-wave is followed by the y descent (opening of the tricuspid valve). The a-wave is large in tricuspid stenosis, pulmonary stenosis, and pulmonary hypertension from any cause. It is absent in atrial fibrillation. Cannon a-waves are giant a-waves which occur when there is atrial contraction against a closed tricuspid valve. It is seen in ventricular ectopics, ventricular tachycardia, complete atrioventricular dissociation, and atrioventricular nodal re-entrant tachycardia.

The c-wave is invisible. The v-wave is large in tricuspid regurgitation. The x descent is prominent in tamponade and pericardial constriction. The y descent is rapid and prominent in constriction (Friedreich's sign) but is absent in tamponade.

Answer 16

D Multiple ventricular ectopics.

See Answer 15 for explanation. Note in electromechanical dissociation there is no effective atrial or ventricular contraction.

Answer 17

A Account for more than 50% of all ASDs.

Ostium secundum ASD accounts for 60% of all ASDs, ostium primum for 30%, and sinus venosus defects for 10%. The left to right shunt across the atria leads to a large increase in pulmonary flow, eventually resulting in pulmonary hypertension and RVH. The increased flow to the right heart is clinically manifest as a middiastolic flow murmur across the tricuspid valve and an ejection systolic murmur across the pulmonary valve. Equalization of pressures on both sides leads to fixed splitting of the second heart sound.

Patients with secundum defects typically present in the third or fourth decades. Recurrent chest infections, breathlessness on exertion, and palpitations due to supraventricular arrhythmias, particularly AF, are common. There is a higher incidence of sinus node disease. Associations include Holt–Oram syndrome (triphalangeal thumbs), MVP, and mitral stenosis (Leutembacher's syndrome). The ECG demonstrates RAD and partial RBBB. Long PR interval is a feature of ostium primum ASD and complete AV canal. Surgery is recommended between ages 5 and 10 years. In older patients surgery should only be performed if the left to right shunt is more than 1.5.

Ostium primum ASD is associated with mitral and tricuspid regurgitation of varying degrees. It is very common in Down's syndrome and also occurs in Kleinfelter's and Noonan's syndromes. Associated renal and splenic abnormalities may be present. It presents in early childhood with features of heart failure. Classic ECG changes include left axis deviation, partial RBBB, RVH, and increased PR interval.

Answer 18

B Slurred R-wave.

WPW has an incidence of 1.5 per 1000. It is more common in males and is due to an accessory pathway between the atria and ventricles (bundle of Kent). The ECG is associated with a short PR interval because the AV node is bypassed during antegrade (atria–ventricle) conduction. Due to early excitation of the ventricle, the QRS has a slurred R-wave (delta wave) and is widened.

Type A WPW = positve delta wave in V1= left sided pathway,
Type B WPW= negative delta wave in V1= right sided pathway.

Palpitations occur in over 60% of patients and are due to AVRT in 70%, atrial flutter in 5%, and atrial fibrillation in 10%. The arrhythmia is usually narrow complex but occasionally may be conducted with bundle branch block. Patients with atrial fibrillation are at risk of sudden death because the accessory pathway can facilitate atrial conduction to the ventricles allowing ventricular fibrillation. These patients should be studied electrophysiologically with a view to ablation of the accessory pathway.

Associations include mitral valve prolapse, HCM, thyrotoxicosis, ASD (secundum), and Ebstein's anomaly (right sided pathway). Management of acute AVRT is with IV adenosine. Recurrent AVRT may be treated with flecainide, propafenone, disopyramide, sotalol, or amiodarone. Digoxin and verapamil are contraindicated because they slow conduction across the AV node but precipitate fast anterograde conduction across the accessory pathway.

Question 19 The following statement is incorrect in WPW syndrome:

A A dominant R-wave in V1 is suggestive of a right sided pathway.
B Atrial flutter is a recognized tachyarrhythmia.
C Patients with atrial fibrillation are at risk of sudden death.
D Is associated with hypertrophic cardiomyopathy.
E A right sided pathway may be associated with Ebstein's anomaly.

Question 20 Adenosine:

A Has a half-life of 30 seconds.
B Is never effective in the termination of ventricular tachycardia.
C Terminates <20% of cases of supraventricular tachycardia.
D Should be used with caution in chronic obstructive airways disease.
E Main site of action is the sino-atrial node.

Question 21 The first heart sound:

A May be soft in WPW.
B May be loud in rheumatic fever.
C Is loud in bradycardia.
D Is variable in atrial flutter.
E May be split in a patient with a cardiac pacemaker.

Answer 19

A A dominant R-wave in V1 is suggestive of a right sided pathway.

See explanations above in Answer 18.

Answer 20

D Should be used with caution in chronic obstructive airways disease.

Adenosine is a purine nucleotide with a half-life of 10–20 seconds. It is effective in the termination of over 90% of SVTs and may also terminate right ventricular outflow tract tachycardia. It may transiently slow down atrial flutter and fibrillation but does not terminate these arrhythmias. It is given intravenously. The main site of action is the atrioventricular node although it does have a slowing down effect on the sinus node. Side-effects include: flushing, dyspnoea, nausea, and bronchospasm. Treatment may be associated with a transient pause on the ECG. It is contraindicated in sick sinus node disease and 2nd and 3rd AV block. It should be used with caution in airways disease including asthma. Its effects are potentiated by dipyridamole and negated by aminophylline.

Answer 21

E May be split in a patient with a cardiac pacemaker.

The first heart sound is:
Loud in:
- Mitral stenosis.
- Tachycardia.
- Short PR interval.

Soft in:
- Mitral regurgitation.
- Long PR interval.
- Anything which causes delayed ventricular contraction, e.g. aortic stenosis.
- MI.

Variable in:
- Atrial fibrillation.
- AV dissociation.
- AVNRT.
- Ventricular tachycardia.

Split in:
- LBBB/RBBB.
- VT.

Note: in WPW the PR interval is short therefore the first heart sound may be loud. In rheumatic heart fever the PR interval may be prolonged producing a soft first sound. Patients with pacemakers conduct with RBBB which may cause the first heart sound to be split.

Question 22 The second heart sound:

A Is soft in hypertension.
B Is widely split in LBBB.
C Demonstrates fixed splitting in ASD.
D Demonstrates reversed splitting in pulmonary hypertension.
E Demonstrates wide splitting in WPW type B.

Question 23 The following is not associated with dissection of the aorta:

A Aortic atherosclerosis.
B Ehler–Danlos syndrome.
C Pregnancy.
D Hypertension in the black population.
E Turner's syndrome.

Question 24 The following statement about infective endocarditis is incorrect:

A Blood cultures are the choice of investigations.
B The absence of vegetations on echocardiography excludes endocarditis.
C May occur in one-third of patients with a normal heart.
D Janeway lesions are a recognized feature.
E Sudden blindness may occur.

Question 25 The following statement about digoxin is incorrect:

A Acts by inhibiting the Na^+/K^+ ATPase.
B Increases the refractory period of the AV node.
C Has inotropic properties.
D Toxicity may be precipitated by hypercalcaemia.
E Its effects are potentiated by concomitant therapy with antacids.

Answer 22

C Demonstrates fixed splitting in ASD.

The second heart sound is:
Normally split:
- During inspiration.

Widely split in:
- RBBB.
- Pulmonary stenosis.
- Pulmonary hypertension.
- VSD/MR (both cause early closure of aortic valve).

Reversed split in:
- LBBB.
- Aortic stenosis.
- Type B WPW (early closure of pulmonary valve).

Fixed split in:
- ASD.

Loud in:
- Hypertension and tachycardia.

Answer 23

A Aortic atherosclerosis.

Causes of aortic dissection include:
- Hypertension (particularly negroid HT).
- Coarctation of the aorta.
- Marfan's syndrome.
- Ehler–Danlos syndrome.
- Noonan's syndrome.
- Turner's syndrome.
- Pregnancy.

Note: syphilis and atherosclerosis do not cause dissection. Classification: Shumway Type A (proximal) and Type B (distal).
- Pathology is cystic medial necrosis.
- More common in males than females.
- Age 40–70 years.
- Frequently fatal: 50% dead in 48 h, 70% in 1 week and 90% in 3 months.
- Proximal dissections may be complicated by aortic regurgitation and tamponade.
- Involvement of the origins of the carotids, left subclavian, and descending aorta may cause neurological deficit, upper limb paralysis, and ischaemia (mesenteric ischaemia, renal failure, and ischaemia to the lower limbs), respectively.

Answer 24

B The absence of vegetations on echocardiography excludes endocarditis.

Infective endocarditis is most commonly due to *Streptococci viridans* (50% of causes on native valves and 10% of all causes on prosthetic valves). In prosthetic valves *Staphylococcus aureus* accounts for the majority (50% of cases). Other bacteria which cause endocarditis include Enterococci and Gram-negative agents. There is an association with *Streptococcus faecalis* endocarditis and carcinoma of the colon.

One-third of cases occur on normal valves. Vegetations <3 mm will not be detected on echocardiography, therefore a normal echo does not exclude the condition. Blood cultures are positive in over 90% of cases. Culture negative endocarditis may occur due to prior treatment with antibiotics, *Coxiella burnetti*, brucellosis, and fungal endocarditis.

Associations include clubbing, Osler's nodes, splinter haemorrhages, Janeway lesions, splenomegaly (30%), Roth spots, mycotic aneurysms and emboli (central retinal artery embolus may cause sudden blindness as in this particular question), and nephritis.

Answer 25

E Its effects are potentiated by concomitant therapy with antacids.

Digoxin is a ouabain derivative which acts by inhibiting the Na^+/K^+ ATPase. The greater influx of sodium resulting from this displaces myocardial cellular calcium, which increases the refractory period of the AVN and has an inotropic effect. Digoxin is effective in the management of established atrial fibrillation and is used as an inotrope in CCF. Toxicity occurs with electrolyte disturbances and concomitant drug therapy.

Tutorial

Causes of digoxin toxicity:
Electrolyte disturbances:
- Hypokalaemia.
- Hypomagnesaemia.
- Hypercalcaemia.

Drugs:
- Quinidine/captopril (reduce renal clearance).
- Amiodarone, verapamil, nifedipine (displace from protein-binding sites).
- Erythromycin/tetracycline (reduce conversion of dihydrodigoxin in the gastrointestinal tract).

Other causes of toxicity:
- Renal failure.
- Hypothyroidism.

Side-effects:
- Nausea, vomiting, anorexia, diarrhoea, gynaecomastia, impotence, xanthopsia, and atrial and ventricular arrhythmias.

ECG changes:
- ST segment depression in 'reverse tick fashion' is not necessarily a feature of toxicity.

Drugs negating the effects of digoxin:
- Antacids/cimetidine (reduce absorption).
- Phenytoin/rifampicin (increase hepatic metabolism).
- Neomycin/sulphasalazine (reduce gut absorption).

Question 26 The following statement is against the diagnosis of pericardial constriction in a patient with swollen ankles:

A A raised JVP.
B There is a prominent x and y descent on the JVP.
C A prior history of chest radiotherapy.
D The presence of pulsus alternans.
E A fall in blood pressure exceeding 10 mmHg (1.3 kPa) during inspiration.

Question 27 The following is true in atrial myxoma:

A Is commoner in males than females.
B Most commonly arises from the interatrial septum.
C Commonly presents with atrial fibrillation.
D Pyrexia is a recognized feature.
E Is associated with a loud fourth heart sound.

Question 28 In Fallot's tetralogy:

A The murmur is due to VSD.
B Right ventricular outflow tract obstruction may worsen with age.
C Pulmonary hypertension is recognized.
D The second heart sound is split.
E A third heart sound is common.

Question 29 The following drug is prognostically important in heart failure:

A Frusemide.
B Digoxin.
C Candesartan.
D Hydralazine.
E Atenolol.

Answer 26

D The presence of pulsus alternans.

Pericardial constriction may be complicated by any form of pericarditis but characteristically occurs in TB, connective tissue diseases, radiotherapy, post-cardiac surgery, bacterial pericarditis, neoplastic infiltration, and chronic renal failure.

Both the LVEDP and RVEDP are equal (and so are the atrial pressures) because both ventricles are equally affected; however, clinical features of right ventricular failure are predominant. Patients classically present with ascites, ankle oedema, and fatigue. Abdominal pain and dyspepsia may be present due to hepatic congestion. The JVP is elevated and paradoxically rises on inspiration (Kussmaul's sign) because blood is drawn into the right ventricle which has limited capacity to expand. The JVP demonstrates prominent x and y descents. There is pulsus paradoxus (a misnomer because what really happens is an exaggeration of what would normally happen, i.e. the blood pressure drops >10 mmHg (1.3 kPa) during inspiration. In normal patients blood pressure also drops during inspiration but not >10 mmHg (1.3 kPa). Symptoms and signs of left heart failure are rare but may occur once atrial pressures exceed 15 mmHg (2 kPa).

Answer 27

D Pyrexia is a recognized feature.

Atrial myxomas are rare. They are almost always benign and 75% arise from the left atrium in the fossa ovalis. The female to male ratio is approximately 2:1. They are usually slow growing polyploid masses which present with:

- Progressive breathlessness, orthopnoea.
- Embolic phenomena.
- Syncopal episodes.
- Constitutional features (25%) such as weight loss, fever, joint pains, malaise (may simulate lymphoma, TB, endocarditis, or vasculitis).

Clinically left atrial myxoma mimics mitral stenosis. However, the opening snap is absent and there in an additional sound in early diastole (tumour plop). Patients with atrial myxoma do not have a loud fourth heart sound unless there is co-existing left ventricular dysfunction. In contrast with mitral stenosis, atrial fibrillation is relatively uncommon. Clubbing is present in <10% of cases. Treatment is with surgical resection and the recurrence rate is 10%.

The ESR is high in the majority. Hypergammaglobulinaemia, leucocytosis, thrombocytopenia, haemolytic anaemia, and polycythaemia are all recognized.

Answer 28

B Right ventricular outflow tract obstruction may worsen with age.

Fallot's tetralogy comprises of large VSD with right to left shunt:

- Pulmonary stenosis.
- Right ventricular hypertrophy.
- Overriding aorta.

Patients present in very early infancy (<9 months) with cyanosis, cardiac failure, and failure to thrive. Clinically there is clubbbing, cyanosis, a right ventricular heave, and an ejection systolic murmur from pulmonary stenosis. The VSD is too large to cause a murmur. The second heart sound is single due to pulmonary stenosis. Pulmonary stenosis protects from pulmonary hypertension.

Recognized symptoms include syncope, palpitation, exertional dyspnoea, and easy fatigue. Complications include secondary polycythaemia and hyperviscosity, endocarditis, paradoxical embolism, and cerebral abscess. Radical sugery is carried out in the first 3–5 years of life. Right ventricular outflow obstruction may worsen with age in the first 3 years of life.

Answer 29

C Candesartan.

The prognosis of heart failure has been improved significantly by drugs inhibiting the renin–angiotensin–aldosterone system and those negating the effects of circulating catecholamines. These drugs include angiotensin converting enzyme inhibitors, angiotensin II receptor blockers such as candesartan, spironolactone, epleronone, and beta-blockers. Three beta-blockers have been shown (in large trials) to improve prognosis in heart failure, notably metoprolol, bisoprolol and carvedilol. Atenolol has not been evaluated in the management of heart failure. Whereas diuretics such as frusemide are effective in improving symptoms secondary to volume overload, they do not improve prognosis. Similarly, hydralazine and isosorbide nitrate in combination have been shown to be as effective as ACE inhibitors with respect to improving symptoms, but these drugs do not alter prognosis. Digoxin is associated with symptomatic improvement through its inotropic effects in patients in atrial fibrillation and sinus rhythm but does not have a positive effect in terms of prognosis.

3 Clinical Pharmacology

Question 1 The following drug is safe safe in breast feeding:

A Chloramphenicol.
B Androgens.
C Carbamazepine.
D Paracetamol.
E Benzodiazepines.

Question 2 Hypothyroidism may be caused by:

A Aminoglycosides.
B Oral contraceptives.
C Lithium.
D Phenytoin.
E Propranolol.

Question 3 Symptoms of asthma may not be exacerbated by:

A Digoxin.
B Propranolol.
C Isocynates.
D Salicylates.
E Sodium cromoglycate.

Answer 1

C Carbamazepine.

Chloroquine is secreted into the breast milk but the amount is too small to be of harm. Carbamazepine, sodium valproate, and phenytoin are also secreted in breast milk but are regarded as being safe. Phenobarbitone, however, should be avoided as it may inhibit the infant's suckling reflex.

Chloramphenicol may cause marrow toxicity in the infant. Androgens cause masculinization of the female infant and precocious puberty in the male. Benzodiazepines cause lethargy and weight loss in the infant.

Tutorial

The following drugs should be avoided in breast-feeding:

Antibiotics:
- Tetracyclines (cause discolouration of the teeth).
- Sulphonamides (kernicterus in jaundiced infants).
- Chloramphenicol.
- Metronidazole.
- Aminoglycosides.
- Isoniazid (rifampicin need not be avoided).
- Cytotoxic drugs.
- High-dose steroid.
- Theophylline (irritability in the infant).

Anticoagulants:
- Phenindiones increase the risk of haemorrhage which is increased by vitamin K deficiency.

Sedatives:
- Chlorpromazine.
- Narcotic analgesics.
- Benzodiazepines.

Drugs that suppress lactation:
- Bromocriptine.
- Frusemide.
- Oestrogens.

Answer 2

C Lithium.

Amiodarone is heavily iodinated resulting in iodine toxicity. The excessive uptake of iodine by the thyroid gland may result in inhibition of thyroid hormone synthesis resulting in hypothyroidism (Wolff–Chaikoff effect), occurring in up to 10% of patients, or excessive thyroid hormone production and hyperthyroidism (Jod–Basedow effect).

The oral contraceptive causes an increase in the thyroid binding globulin (TBG) resulting in an increase in the total T3 and T4 without affecting free hormone concentrations. Similarly, androgens reduce TBG and hence total T3 and T4.

Lithium is a well-recognized cause of iatrogenic hypothyroidism and, as with iodides, it is most likely to have this effect in patients who have underlying thyroid disease.

Phenytoin has several effects. These include:
- Inhibition of the binding of thyroid hormone to TBG resulting in a reduction in T4 levels without changes in serum TSH.
- Increased cellular uptake and metabolism of T4. (Phenobarbitone shares this effect.)
- Patients taking phenytoin are metabolically euthyroid.
- Patients who are taking thyroxine for hypothyroidism and phenytoin will require higher doses of thyroxine for the above reason.

Propranolol reduces T4 to T3 deiodination in the liver and kidneys.

Propylthyouracil and corticosteroids also have this effect. Iodate and amiodarone reduce intrapituitary conversion of T4 to T3.

Answer 3

A Digoxin.

Nonselective beta-blockers such as propranolol block the β2 receptors causing bronchoconstriction. Unfortunately selective beta-blockers often produce this effect as well, but to a milder extent.

Isocynates are an important cause of occupational asthma. Salicylates inhibit arachidonic acid metabolism via the cyclooxygenase pathway preventing the synthesis of prostaglandins. The arachidonic acid is then metabolized by the lipooxygenase pathway resulting in the production of leukotrienes which are mediators of anaphylaxis.

Although sodium cromoglycate is useful as a prophylactic agent in exercise-induced asthma, inhalation of the powder precipitates bronchospasm in some individuals.

Question 4 The following is not true for a female aged 40 years taking the oral contraceptive:

A She should be advised against this if she is known to have gall stones.
B The maternal mortality in a woman her age is several times greater than the risk of thromboembolism.
C A woman of her age should not be taking such medication.
D The pill may cause disturbance of her liver function tests.
E There may be a disturbance in her carbohydrate metabolism.

Question 5 The following drug is safe in mild renal impairment:

A Azathioprine.
B Aminoglycosides.
C Enalapril.
D Lithium.
E Gentamicin.

Answer 4

C A woman of her age should not be taking such medication.

Gall bladder disease is a relative contraindication for using the pill. Other relative contraindications include hypertension and ischaemic heart disease.

Steroid oral contraceptives are metabolized by the liver and for this reason they may affect the metabolism of carbohydrates, lipids, plasma proteins, amino acids, vitamins, and clotting factors. Benign hepatic adenoma is an uncommon consequence of the combined oral contraceptive. Glucose intolerance is a recognized side-effect which may be exacerbated by obesity and smoking.

For this age group the maternal morbidity and mortality risks from pregnancy are greater than those from thromboembolism, provided that all contra-indications for prescription are taken into account prior to starting treatment. The combined pill is associated with a threefold increase in venous thromboembolism. This risk is unaffected by age, smoking, or duration of pill use, but is higher in obese women and those with a history of pregnancy-induced hypertension.

Tutorial

Absolute contraindications for taking the combined OCP include:

- Ischaemic heart disease, cardiomyopathy, and most types of cardiac valvular disease.
- Venous thrombosis or known predisposition to thrombosis.
- Cerebrovascular disease, vascular malformations in the brain.
- Pulmonary hypertension.
- Hyperlipidaemia.
- Active liver disease, recurrent cholestasis, liver tumour.
- Porphyria.
- Pregnancy and undiagnosed genital bleeding.
- Severe hypertension.
- Hormone dependent tumours of the breast, endometrium, kidney, and malignant melanoma.

The main side-effects of the OCP are due to the oestrogens. Progesterone is responsible for weight gain, acne, oedema, and break-through bleeding.

Side-effects

Metabolic side-effects include:

- Impaired glucose tolerance.
- An increase in the serum cholesterol and triglycerides.
- The precipitation of porphyria in susceptible individuals.

Vascular side-effects:

- Hypertension.
- Venous thrombosis.
- CVA/MI.

Drug interactions

Enzyme-inducing drugs may reduce the contraceptive protection of the OCP. These drugs are:

- Anticonvulsants (phenytoin, carbamazepine, phenobarbitone).
- Rifampicin, isoniazid.
- Griseofulvin.
- Benzodiazepines.

Answer 5

A Azathioprine.

Frusemide is safe. Azathioprine should be avoided in severe renal impairment. Aminoglycosides have an increased risk of producing nephrotoxicity and ototoxicity even in mild renal impairment. The dose should be reduced.

Short-acting ACE inhibitors such as captopril are safe but the dose of long-acting ACE inhibitors should be reduced. Potassium sparing diuretics should be avoided to prevent hyperkalaemia.

Tutorial

Drugs that are metabolized or excreted mainly by the kidney accumulate in renal impairment.

Drugs that can be used in normal doses include:
Antibiotics:
- Cloxacillin.
- Chloramphenicol.
- Erythromycin.

Cardiac drugs:
- Thiazide diuretics and loop diuretics.
- Calcium antagonists.
- Clonidine.
- Hydralazine.
- Opiates.
- Wafarin.
- Phenindione.
- Steroids.

Drugs requiring dose adjustment in renal impairment include:
Antibiotics:
- Penicillin G.
- Aminoglycosides.
- Vancomycin.
- Sulphonamides.
- Metronidazole.
- Cephalosporins.

Cardiovascular drugs:
- Digoxin.
- Methyldopa.
- ACE inhibitors.
- Flecainide.

Diabetic drugs:
- Sulphonylureas.
- Insulin.

Drugs to be avoided in renal impairment:
Antibiotics:
- Tetracyclines.
- Nitrofurantoin.
- Amphotericin B.

Cardiac drugs:
- Potassium sparing diuretics.
- Potassium supplements.
- NSAIDs.
- Lithium.

Question 6 Obstructive jaundice is not a recognized side-effect of:

A Chlorpromazine.
B Carbimazole.
C Azithromycin.
D Methyldopa.
E Methyl testosterone.

Question 7 The following drug is safe in liver failure:

A ACE inhibitors.
B Methotrexate.
C Warfarin.
D Tetracycline.
E Theophylline.

Question 8 The following statement is not true:

A Paracetamol has analgesic but little or no anti-inflammatory effect in man.
B Buffered aspirin causes intestinal bleeding.
C Necrotizing papillitis occurs as a result of dihydrocodeine administration.
D Colchicine has no uricosuric effect.
E Acetozolamide may cause renal tubular acidosis.

Answer 6

D Methyldopa.

Cholestatic jaundice is a recognized side-effect of a number of drugs and these should be avoided in patients with underlying liver disease. For the MRCP Part 1 the following drugs are favourites for causing either biochemical or frank obstructive jaundice:

Antibiotics:
- Erythromycin estolate, azithromycin (40%).
- Flucloxacillin.
- Sulphonamides.

Anti-TB:
- Rifampicin.
- Isoniazid.

Hormones:
- Oral contraceptives.
- Androgens (e.g. methyl testosterone).
- Synthetic anabolic steroids.

Phenothiazines (e.g. chlorpromazine [2%]).

Antithyroid drugs (e.g. carbimazole).

Hypoglycaemic drugs (e.g. chlorpropamide [25%]).

TCAs.

NSAIDs.

Metformin should be avoided in liver impairment due to an increased risk of lactic acidosis. It is the sulphonylurea oral hypoglycaemics that cause obstructive jaundice. Methyldopa causes hepatitis.

Answer 7

A ACE inhibitors.

Warfarin and theophylline are metabolized in the liver, and therefore have increased risk of toxicity in liver impairment. Methotrexate is hepatotoxic. ACE inhibitors should be used with caution in renal disease. Rarely, they can cause deranged LFTs and even cholestasis but they are said to be safe in existing liver disease. Lithium is excreted mainly by the kidneys and again is safe in liver disease, but it should be used with caution in renal disease.

Tutorial

Other drugs metabolized by the liver include:
- Phenytoin.
- Corticosteroids.
- Narcotic analgesics.
- Phenothiazines.
- Barbiturates.

Other drugs to be avoided in liver disease:
- NSAIDs – cause fluid retention.
- Sedatives – may precipitate encephalopathy.
- Hepatotoxic drugs:
  - Methotrexate.
  - Paracetamol.
  - Tetracycline.

Answer 8

C Necrotizing papillitis occurs as a result of dihydrocodeine administration.

Paracetamol has no anti-inflammatory effects. Renal tubular acidosis may be caused by acetozolamide, amphotericin B, and out-of-date tetracyclines. Probenacid and sulphinpyrazone are uricosuric drugs.

Aspirin and other NSAIDs inhibit the enzyme cyclooxygenase and hence the formation of prostaglandins from arachidonate. Buffering makes little difference to this action and the protective action of prostaglandins is hindered, promoting peptic ulceration and gastrointestinal bleeding.

Papillary necrosis is caused by NSAIDs, especially phenacetin.

Question 9 In patients taking monoamine oxidase inhibitors, adverse reactions may occur as a result of ingestion of the following with the exception of:

A Amitriptyline.
B Levodopa.
C Isoprenaline.
D Aspirin.
E Pethidine.

Question 10 An undesirable side-effect of primidone administration is:

A Renal papillary necrosis.
B Insomnia.
C Ataxia.
D Gum hypertrophy.
E Diarrhoea.

Question 11 The following drug combinations may not prove to be beneficial:

A Frusemide and spironolactone.
B Probenecid and indomethacin.
C Benzylpenicillin and cloxacillin.
D Methyldopa and bethanidine.
E Neostigmine and pilocarpine.

Question 12 Phenylbutazone therapy:

A Has no effect on urinary excretion of uric acid.
B May cause pernicious anaemia.
C Needs to be used with caution in congestive cardiac failure.
D May be of use in treating osteoarthritis of the hip.
E Is the first line of treatment of ankylosing spondylitis.

Question 13 The following drug is not uricosuric:

A Phenylbutazone.
B Sulphinpyrazone.
C Colchicine.
D Aspirin.
E Azathioprine.

Answer 9

D Aspirin.

Sympathomimetic amines interact with MAOIs to produce:
- Severe hypertension (hypertensive crisis and subarachnoid haemorrhage).
- CNS excitation.
- Hyperpyrexia.
- Prolonged action of interacting drugs.

Drugs that are contraindicated in patients on MAOIs include:
- Tricyclic antidepressants.
- Amphetamines.
- Pethidine.
- Isoprenaline.
- Levodopa.
- Barbiturates.
- Tyramine-containing foods should also be avoided such as:
  - Mature cheese (cream cheese and cottage cheese do not contain tyramine).
  - Yeast extracts.
  - Red wine and beer.
  - Chicken liver.
  - Broad beans.
  - Coffee.

Answer 10

C Ataxia.

All anticonvulsants act on the CNS and hence can cause ataxia, seizures, mood swings, drowsiness, confusion, and tremor. In toxicity visual disturbances and agitation are common. Most of these drugs also cause Stevens–Johnson syndrome.

Anticonvulsants frequently feature in the MRCP Part 1. The following should cover the essential points with reference to previous questions:

- Ethosuximide is still the drug of choice in petit mal seizures.
- Phenytoin can be used for all sorts of seizures except petit mal. It can also be used to treat trigeminal neuralgia.
- Important nonCNS side-effects of phenytoin include:
  - Coarse facies, acne, gum hypertrophy, and hirsutism.
  - Lymphadenopathy and peripheral neuropathy.
  - Megaloblastic anaemia and osteomalacia.
  - Hepatitis (avoid in hepatic impairment) and SLE syndrome.

Carbamazepine is used in preference to phenytoin in trigeminal neuralgia. Important side-effects are SIADH, cholestatic jaundice, constipation, and alopecia. Lamotrigine is a second line drug. It causes the entire spectrum of CNS side-effects as well as angioedema.

Answer 11

E Neostigmine and pilocarpine.

Spironolactone should not be used with other potassium sparing diuretics such as amiloride or ACE inhibitors due to risk of hyperkalaemia.

Aspirin antagonizes the uricosuric effect of probenecid and indeed promotes the retention of urate thereby increasing the risk of acute gout. One of the most important aspects of managing gout is to withdraw drugs that increase the plasma uric acid such as aspirin and thiazide diuretics.

Probenecid can be used with allopurinol in the management of chronic gout. Probenecid reduces the excretion of a number of drugs resulting in an increased risk of toxicity. It should be used with caution with:
- Indomethacin.
- Cephalosporins, penicillins.
- Acyclovir, zidovudine.
- Methotrexate.

Neostigmine is an anticholinesterase and therefore prolongs the action of acetylcholine. It is used to enhance neuromuscular transmission in voluntary and involuntary muscles in myasthenia gravis.

Answer 12

C Needs to be used with caution in congestive cardiac failure.

Phenylbutazone is uricosuric. It may cause fluid retention and hence needs to be used with caution in CCF. It is used in ankylosing spondylitis when other treatments have failed and is not used to treat osteoarthritis. It may cause a variety of haematological side-effects including leucopenia, thrombocytopenia, agranulocytosis, and aplastic anaemia. Other important side-effects are:

- Pulmonary syndrome: fever and dyspnoea.
- Aggravation of SLE.
- Hepatitis.
- Erythema multiforme.

Answer 13

C Colchicine.

Uricosuric drugs increase the excretion of uric acid in the urine. They should never be used to treat an acute attack of gout. Instead, acute attacks are treated with colchicine or NSAIDs.

The main uricosuric drugs in terms of treatment of gout are probenecid and sulphinpyrazone. Aspirin is uricosuric in high doses. At low doses it reduces uric acid excretion. Azapropazone and phenylbutazone also have a uricosuric effect. The former may be useful in the long-term treatment of chronic gout.

Allopurinol has no uricosuric effects. It is useful in cases of renal impairment. It is converted into an active metabolite with a long half-life. Allopurinol should not be used until the acute attack has completely subsided as further attacks may be precipitated.

Drugs known to reduce uric acid excretion and promote gout include:

- Loop and thiazide diuretics.
- Ethambutol.
- Pyrazinamide.
- Low-dose salicylates.
- Cytotoxics.

Question 14 The following is not true of phenytoin sodium:

A Can be used to control grand mal seizures when used alone.
B Reduces the metabolism of tiagabine.
C May produce hirsutism in girls.
D Is superior to ethosuximide in petit mal seizures.
E May cause ataxia.

Answer 14

D Is superior to ethosuximide in petit mal seizures.

Covered in Answer 10.

Tiagabine is a fairly recent antiepileptic drug licensed as adjunctive therapy in the UK.

Tutorial

More recent drug treatments for epilepsy:

Vigabatrin

Vigabatrin was licensed in 1989 as an add-on therapy for partial seizures with or without secondary generalization, and as a monotherapy for infantile spasms. It can worsen myoclonic epilepsies and generalized absences. It acts by irreversibly inhibiting the enzyme responsible for the breakdown of GABA which is the major inhibitory neurotransmitter in the brain. The half-life of the drug itself is short at 5–7 hours, and is excreted by the kidneys.

It interacts with phenytoin, reducing the concentration by 20–30%.

Side-effects consist of sedation, fatigue, headache, dizziness, weight gain, and depression. The drug should be withdrawn immediately if the patient complains of agitation or develops a thought disorder, and should be avoided in patients with a psychiatric history.

Lamotrigine

Lamotrigine was licensed in 1991 as adjunctive treatment and monotherapy for partial and tonic–clonic seizures, and it may also be used for seizures associated with the Lennox–Gastaut syndrome. It is also effective in generalized absences and myoclonc jerks. It acts by stabilizing the presynaptic neuronal membranes by prolonging the slow inactivated state of the voltage dependent sodium channels. It is metabolized to an inactive conjugate in the liver and its elimination half-life is 22–36 hours.

It does not influence the metabolism of any other antiepileptic. Enzyme-inducing antiepileptics such as phenytoin and carbamazepine, however, accelerate the metabolism of lamotrigine to around 15 hours, whereas enzyme inhibitors such as sodium valproate prolong its half-life to about 60 hours. Patients who are already being treated with carbamazepine often develop headache, dizziness, ataxia, and diplopia when lamotrigine is introduced and should be warned of this interaction.

Side-effects of lamotrigine consist of headache, dizziness, ataxia, tremor, diplopia, and sedation. This drug can cause a fever, associated with arthralgia, myalgia, lymphadenopathy, eosinophilia, and maculopapular rash (3–5%). It can also cause Stevens–Johnson or Lyell's syndrome.

Gabapentin

Gabapentin was licensed in 1993 for add-on treatment in patients with partial seizures, with or without secondary generalization. Its mechanism of action is thought to be by binding to calcium channels in the brain. It has a half-life of 4–7 hours and is excreted unchanged by the kidneys.

Side-effects include somnolence, dizziness, ataxia, fatigue, tremor, and nystagmus. It also causes vomiting, flatulence, diarrhoea, and myoclonic jerking.

Topiramide

Topiramide was licensed in 1995 as an add-on therapy for refractory partial epilepsy with or without secondary generalization. It has also been effective in the treatment of idiopathic epilepsy. It acts by blocking sodium channels, attenuating neuronal excitation, and enhances GABA-mediated inhibition.

Phenytoin and carbamazepine induce the metabolism of topiramide, reducing its effectiveness by up to 40%. Topiramide may also accelerate the metabolism of phenytoin and the oestrogenic component of the oral contraceptive.

Side-effects consist of poor concentration, word finding difficulty, dysarthria, ataxia, paraesthesia, and somnolence.

Tiagabine

Tiagabine was licenced in 1998 as adjunctive therapy. It controls partial seizures with or without secondary generalization. It acts by inhibiting the uptake of GABA into neurones. It has a short half-life of 4–9 hours and it does not alter the plasma concentration of other antiepileptic drugs. Its own metabolism is accelerated by phenytoin and carbamazepine. It should be taken with food to avoid high peak concentrations and dizziness.

Side-effects consist of dizziness, asthenia, nervousness, depression, and diarrhoea.

Question 15 The following is not true for digoxin toxicity:

A May be precipitated by hypokalaemia.
B Is not due to an idiosyncratic reaction to the drug.
C Is less likely to occur in the elderly.
D May cause paroxysmal atrial fibrillation.
E May be aggravated by hypercalcaemia.

Question 16 Fast acetylators will show a diminished response to the following drug:

A Digoxin.
B Isoniazid.
C Dapsone.
D Nitrazepam.
E Procainamide.

Question 17 The syndrome of inappropriate antidiuretic hormone secretion may not be caused by:

A Chlorpropamide.
B Demeclocycline.
C Carbamazepine.
D Thiazide diuretics.
E Opiates.

Answer 15

C Is less likely to occur in the elderly.

The elderly are most prone to digoxin toxicity. Digoxin can cause a variety of arrhythmias including atrial tachycardia, flutter and fibrillation, ventricular extrasystoles, and bigeminy.

An idiosyncratic reaction is an unexpected and unusual sensitivity exhibited by an individual to a particular drug. This is definitely not the case with digoxin.

Tutorial

Factors increasing the risks of digoxin toxicity:
- Hypokalaemia.
- Hypercalcaemia.
- Hypomagnesaemia.
- Drug interactions with quinidine, amiodarone, verapamil, and beta-blockers which reduce the renal excretion of digoxin.
- Renal failure.
- Hypoxia.

Symptoms of toxicity:
- Anorexia, nausea, and vomiting.
- Confusion.
- Insomnia.
- Xanthopsia (yellow vision).

Answer 16

A Digoxin.

Fast acetylation is inherited as an autosomal recessive trait. Their response to the following drugs will be diminished:
- Hydralazine.
- Isoniazid.
- Dapsone.
- Nitrazepam.
- Procainamide.

Slow acetylators may develop a lupus-like syndrome on the above medication.

Tutorial

Drug-induced lupus is dose related and usually reversible. Patients are ANF-positive, but renal and central nervous system involvement seldom occurs. It is more frequent in subjects with HLA DR4. Serum complement is usually unaffected.

Suxamethonium sensitivity due to abnormal plasma pseudocholinesterase is another example of genetic variation in drug metabolism. In normal individuals it has a 5 minute duration of action and is hence ideal for endotracheal intubation. It mimics acetylcholine at the neuromuscular junction causing neuromuscular blockade and paralysis which is rapid and short-lived. Patients with abnormal pseudocholinesterase show prolonged apnoea and muscle paralysis when anaesthetized with suxamethonium, due to delayed degradation.

Answer 17

B Demeclocycline.

Thiazides cause SIADH and may be used to treat nephrogenic diabetes insipidus. Carbamazepine and clofibrate cause SIADH and may be used to treat partial cranial diabetes insipidus.

Other drugs causing SIADH include:
- Morphine.
- Chlorpropamide.
- Rifampicin.
- Cyclophosphamide and vincristine.

Demeclocycline and lithium cause nephrogenic diabetes insipidus. Demeclocycline may be used to treat SIADH.

Question 18 Penicillamine:

A Is not effective in the treatment of rheumatoid vasculitis.
B Maximum response to treatment occurs in the first 3 months.
C May cause loss of taste.
D Does not cause chronic active hepatitis.
E May cause Wilson's disease.

Question 19 The following are liver enzyme inducers with the exception of:

A Valproate.
B Phenytoin.
C Chronic alcohol ingestion.
D Glibenclamide.
E Cimetidine.

Question 20 Peripheral neuropathy is a recognized side-effect of treatment with the following with the exception of:

A Amiodarone.
B Ethambutol.
C Metronidazole.
D Chlorpropamide.
E Chlorpromazine.

Answer 1

E Eruptive xanthomata.

Granuloma annulare typically occurs over a bony prominence and most commonly on the dorsum of the hand. It consists of flesh coloured papules which coalesce to form an annular pattern. The lesion may also affect the wrists, ankles, and feet. It may also occur in cases of impaired glucose tolerance and is not related to glycaemic control. Eruptive xanthomata are due to hypertriglyceridaemia seen in poorly controlled diabetes. They also occur in hyperlipoproteinaemias (hereditary and that occurring secondary to hypothyroidism and nephrotic syndrome).

Scleroedema occurs in diabetics, sclerodactyly is a manifestation of scleroderma. Erythema nodosum and Stevens–Johnson syndrome do not occur as a result of diabetes.

Tutorial

Other skin disorders occuring in diabetes include:
- Diabetic dermopathy: flat, hyperpigmented, atrophic lesions found most commonly on the shins. The condition is more common in patients who have microangiopathy affecting other organs.
- Necrobiosis lipoidicum: not specific for diabetes and unrelated to glycaemic control.
- Diabetic bullae: more common in patients who have neuropathy.
- Abscesses.
- Boils.
- Carbuncles.

Answer 2

D Acne vulgaris.

Tutorial

Other skin conditions exacerbated by sunlight include:
- Erythema multiforme.
- Darier's disease.
- Pemphigus.
- Psoriasis.
- Atopic dermatitis.
- Senile elastosis.
- Chloasma.

Drugs producing photosensitvity:
- Amiodarone.
- Chlorpromazine
- Thiazide diuretics.
- NSAIDs.
- Quinine.
- Tetracycline.
- Sulphonamides.
- Retinoids.

The following skin conditions may be exacerbated by exposure to sunlight:
- Porphyria cutanea tarda.
- Discoid lupus erythematosis.
- Xeroderma pigmentosum.
- Pellagra.

In the cutaneous porphyrias, porphyrins are deposited in the skin and react with sunlight to produce:
- Blisters.
- Erythema.
- Scarring.
- Hypertrichosis affecting the facial region.
- Thickening of facial skin with loss of hair (pseudo-scleroderma).
- Hyper-/hypopigmentation.
- Itching.

Cutaneous porphyrias include:
- Porpyhria cutanea tarda.
- Variegate porphyria.
- Erythropoetic porphyria.

(Note: acute intermittent porphyria has no cutaneous features.)

Discoid and systemic lupus erythmatosis may be exacerbated by sunlight. Xeroderma pigmentosum is an autosomal dominant condition where there is a defect in DNA repair. It is associated with severe, delayed onset of persistent sunburn and the premature aging of skin, as well as development of melanoma and other skin malignancies. Pellagra is caused by niacin deficiency. It is associated with a photosensive dermatitis characterized by initial erythema, followed by thickening and pigmentation of the skin.

Answer 3

A Behçet's disease.

Tutorial

Other causes of oral and genital lesions include:
- Herpes simplex infection.
- Syphilis.
- Herpangina (Coxsackie virus type A).
- Candidiasis.
- Lichen planus.

Oral ulceration occurs in a 100% of patients with Behçet's disease and genital ulceration in 75%. Other cutaneous manifestations of Behçet's disease include erythema nodosum and superficial migrating thrombophlebitis. Stevens–Johnson syndrome is a severe form of erythema multiforme with lesions occurring in the mouth, conjunctiva, anal, and genital regions.

Lymphogranuloma inguinale is caused by *Chlamydia trachomatis* and is a sexually transmitted disease. It involves the genitals but not the oral cavity. The lesion consists of a painless ulcerating papule associated with tender inguinal lymphadenopathy. The overlying skin develops a dusky erythmatous colouration.

Pityriasis rosea consists of scaling lesions occurring most commonly on the trunk and proximal aspects of the limbs.

Lichen planus is not associated with ulcer formation.

Question 4 When the following conditions develop in or after middle age, internal malignancy must be suspected with the exception of:

A Acanthosis nigricans.
B Xanthoma tuberosum.
C Erythema gyratum repens.
D Dermatomyositis.
E Generalized pruritis.

Question 5 The following is a recognized finding in psoriasis:

A Iridocyclitis.
B Angular stomatitis.
C Dystrophy of the nails.
D Loss of hair.
E Response to chloroquine.

Question 6 The following is true for pityriasis rosea:

A Is a fungal infection.
B Is characterized by flat scaly patches.
C Tends to recur after apparent cure.
D May be preceded by intense itching.
E Is frequently associated with oro-genital ulceration.

Question 7 The following may occur as a result of streptococcal infection:

A Boils.
B Erythema induratum (Bazin's disease).
C Erythema nodosum.
D Acne vulgaris.
E Infantile eczema.

Answer 4

B Xanthoma tuberosum.

Acanthosis nigricans occurs in bowel and bronchial malignancies as well as some lymphomas. Twenty percent of all cases of dermatomyositis are associated with underlying malignancy of the bronchus, breast, stomach, and ovary. In men over the age of 50 years 60% will have carcinoma, most often affecting the bronchus.

Generalized pruritis is common and often severe in the reticuloses (Hodgkin's disease). In this case it is exacerbated by alcohol, but alcohol-induced pain of the lymph nodes is more common. The skin may also become very dry, amounting to ichthyosis.

Dermatomyositis is more common in women. General ill health and fever are common on presentation, and skin involvement occurs in 60% and consists of:

- Heliotrope rash, purple in colouration, around the eyes.
- Violet oedematous lesions over the small joints of the hands with telangiectasia.
- Arteritic lesions around the nails.

Muscle involvement:

- Proximal myopathy.
- Dysphagia.
- Muscle wasting.
- Cardiomyopathy.

The prognosis depends on the underlying cause. In the absence of malignancy the disease may persist with exacerbations and remissions for 10–20 years until death occurs from cardiac or respiratory causes.

Erythema gyratum repens may complicate bronchial carcinoma.

Tutorial

Other cutaneous manifestations of malignancy include:

- Urticaria.
- Tylosis.
- Erythema multiforme.

Answer 5

C Dystrophy of the nails.

In psoriasis, the eyes and mucous membranes are not involved. Nails are affected in 50% of patients who have cutaneous psoriasis, and 90% of patients with psoriatic arthropathy. Nail lesions include:

- Pitting.
- Longitudinal ridges.
- Onycholysis (separation of nail plate from distal nail bed).
- Discolouration.

Alopecia is not a feature. Drugs like chloroquine and lithium exacerbate psoriasis, and chloroquine may precipitate an attack of psoriasis.

Tutorial

Psoriasis has a strong genetic component and is associated with HLA B13, B17, Cw6, B27.

Other conditions known to precipitate and exacerbate psoriasis include:

- Pregnancy.
- Stress.
- Alcohol and cigarette smoking.
- Trauma (Koebner phenomenon).
- Infection (streptococci, HIV).
- Drugs (lithium, antimalarials).
- Sunlight exacerbates psoriasis in up to 10% of cases.

The Koebner phenomenon describes the development of lesions at the site of trauma to the skin.

It occurs in:

- Lichen planus.
- Psoriasis.
- Eczema.
- Viral warts.
- Vitiligo.
- Keloids.
- Sarcoidosis.

Answer 6

B Is characterized by flat scaly patches.

Pityriasis rosea is not a fungal infection and is most probably caused by a virus. The rash itself is preceded by a solitary red, scaly, oval lesion on the trunk or abdomen known as a 'herald patch'. This is followed by a mildly itchy macular rash which may cover the entire trunk, upper thighs, and arms. The macules are oval with peripheral scales and tend to be aligned along natural skin creases and ribs. It usually clears within 6–8 weeks without treatment. The oral and genital mucosa are not affected.

Answer 7

C Erythema nodosum.

Streptococcus pyogenes is a frequent cause of skin infection. In cases of rheumatic fever which follow a streptococcal sore throat, there may be an associated erythematous punctate rash or even a purpuric rash in septicaemia. It is a well recognized cause of erythema nodosum.

Other cutaneous complications include erysipelas which is characterized by the sudden appearance of an erythematous plaque on the face or leg which enlarges peripherally. There is small vesicle and bulla formation at the advancing edges, giving rise to the crusting appearance. It is often accompanied by a systemic febrile illness with regional lymphadenopathy. Recurrent attacks of erysipelas can produce lymphatic obstruction and lymphoedema. Cellulitis can also be caused by this organism.

Question 8 The following condition is likely to present as a bullous eruption:

A Acquired syphilis.
B Mastocytosis.
C Urticaria.
D Phenylketonuria.
E Atopic eczema.

Question 9 Severe pruritis occurs in:

A Dermatitis herpetiformis.
B Sensory neuropathy.
C Psoriasis.
D Tylosis palmaris.
E Molluscum contagiosum.

Question 10 Perforating ulcers in the feet may occur in:

A Diabetes.
B Peripheral vascular disease.
C Rheumatoid arthritis.
D Sarcoidosis.
E Varicose ulceration.

Answer 8

B Mastocytosis.

Congenital syphilis may be associated with a cutaneous bullous eruption in a neonate.

Cutaneous mastocytosis is principally a disorder of childhood. Features include urticaria pigmentosa affecting the trunk and limbs. Trauma to nonaffected skin may demonstrate dermographism. Flushing or skin irritation may follow a change in temperature of surroundings, emotional upset, or drugs that release histamine (aspirin, codeine). The disease remits in children although adult-onset disease does not. It may be congenital, presenting with bullous, blistering skin lesions. In childhood the skin becomes thick and leathery and there may be hepatosplenomegaly in diffuse disease.

Adult disease is associated with telangiectasia of the skin and there may be involvement of the bone marrow and skeletal system. There may also be symptoms of headache, bronchospasm, tachycardia, hypotension, and diarrhoea.

There are three types of epidermolysis bullosa:

- Dystrophica:
  – Type I: autosomal dominant, bullae occur on limbs in infancy.
  – Type II: autosomal recessive, bullae are present at birth with denudation of large areas of skin. There is widespread scarring of the skin with contracture and fusion between the fingers and toes leading to syndactyly.
- Simplex: presents in the first year of life. Blisters occur at areas of contact, e.g. palms and knees. Scarring is unusual. The defect is in the anchoring fibrils of the basal layer cells of the epidermis.
- Letalis (junctional): associated with death in infancy. There are widespread blistering lesions of the skin which fail to heal. The abnormality is within the lamina lucida.

Answer 9

A Dermatitis herpetiformis.

Severe pruritis occurs in dermatitis herpetiformis, which is associated with a papulovesicular rash affecting the extensor surfaces and the very high possibility that the patient has coeliac disease. The mucosal membranes are occasionally affected. IgA deposits are found in the basal lamina of normal skin of these patients and are diagnostic. In most cases the deposits are granular but in up to 20% of patients, they are linear. Coeliac disease occurring in these patients is as a rule less severe and is associated with granular deposits. Treatment of the rash is with dapsone. A gluten-free diet has also been shown to improve skin lesions.

Tutorial

Other dermatological causes of severe pruritis include:

- Mites (scabies, pediculosis).
- Eczema.
- Urticaria.
- Lichen planus.
- Lichen simplex chronicus (a form of eczema characterized by epidermal hyperplasia associated with an itch–scratch cycle).
- Miliaria rubra (prickly heat).
- Thread worms.
- Contact dermatitis, fibre glass dermatitis.

Systemic causes of pruritis:

- Liver disease (due to biliary obstruction) – treatment is with cholestyramine.
- Chronic renal failure (may be secondary to hyperparathyroidism).
- Iron deficiency.
- Polycythaemia rubra vera (itch is triggered by contact with water or due to a sudden fall in skin temperature).
- Hodgkin's disease (often severe and may be exacerbated further by development of ichthyosis).
- Endocrine (hyper-/hypothyroidism, diabetes mellitus, carcinoid).
- Malignancy.
- Parasitic infections (schistosomiasis, trichinosis, onchocerciasis).
- Connective tissue diseases (SLE, scleroderma, sicca syndrome).
- Drugs (cocaine, morphine, allergic drug reactions).

Answer 10

A Diabetes.

Perforating foot ulcers are a feature of diabetes mellitus, leprosy, and syphilis. They are trophic ulcers which occur in an insensitive foot as a result of neuropathic involvement by the disease process.

Question 11 Blisters in the skin do not occur in:

A Epidermolysis bullosa.
B Secondary syphilis.
C Barbiturate overdose.
D Impetigo.
E Necrotizing vasculitis.

Question 12 There is an increased incidence of leg ulceration in the following conditions with the exception of:

A Sickle cell disease.
B Rheumatoid arthritis.
C Klinefelter's syndrome.
D Addison's disease.
E Spina bifida.

Question 13 Changes in the nail bed may be seen in:

A Bacterial endocarditis.
B Primary hypoparathyroidism.
C Psoriasis.
D Severe hypoalbuminaemia.
E Hypothyroidism.

Question 14 Scarring alopecia is not a feature of:

A Lichen planus.
B Alopecia areata.
C Tinea capitis.
D Scleroderma.
E Staphylococcal folliculitis.

Answer 11

B Secondary syphilis.

Epidermolysis bullosa is associated with blister formation, as is drug coma secondary to barbiturate overdose. Impetigo is a blistering eruption affecting the face caused by staphylococcus/streptococcus or a combination of the two. Bullous lesions are less common and occur in infection by staphylococcus strains which also cause toxic epidermal necrolytic vasculitis.

Dermatological causes of blistering lesions:
- Herpes simplex and zoster infections.
- Staphylococcal and streptococcal infections (see above).
- Coxsackie virus infection (hand, foot, and mouth disease) is associated with vesicles and maculopapular eruption on palms and soles. The organism also causes herpangina which is characterized by vesicular eruption in the oropharyngeal region.

Cutaneous disorders:
- Eczema.
- Infiltration (carcinoma, amyloid).

Immunological:
- Bullous pemphigoid.
- Dermatitis herpetiformis.
- Epidermolysis bullosa.
- Porphyria cutanea tarda.
- Lichen planus.

Drugs:
- Barbiturates.
- Aspirin, paracetamol.
- Any drug causing erythema multiforme.

Answer 12

D Addison's disease.

Most leg ulcers have a multifactorial origin of ischaemia, immobility, anaemia, venous hypertension, and infection. Venous ulceration accounts for 60% of all leg ulcers, arterial 10%, mixed venous/arterial 20%, and others 10%.

Patients with sickle cell disease suffer from microinfarctions at many sites including the skin, resulting in ulceration. Rheumatoid arthritis is a vasculitis and causes leg ulceration by a similar mechanism. Patients with Klinefelter's syndrome are prone to venous ulcers. Neuropathy in spina bifida predisposes to leg ulceration.

Tutorial

Other causes of leg ulceration include:
- Lymphatic obstruction, e.g. Milroy's disease.
- Diabetes.
- Tabes dorsalis.
- Leprosy.
- Malignancy especially squamous cell carcinoma.
- Pyoderma gangrenosum.
- As a complication of erysipelas or other streptococcus/staphylococcus infection.
- Trauma.

Answer 13

E Hypothyroidism.

Splinter haemorrhages and clubbing may complicate subacute bacterial endocarditis. Primary hypoparathyroidism may be associated with mucocutaneous candidiasis with nail involvement. Other skin manifestations of this disorder include alopecia and vitiligo.

Nail involvement occurs in up to 90% of patients with psoriasis and is manifested by nail pitting, ribbing (transverse ridging on the dorsal surface), splinter haemorrhages, onycholysis, and subungual hyperkeratosis. Leukonychia (abnormal whiteness at the base of the nails) occurs in conditions associated with severe hypoalbuminaemia, e.g. liver disease.

Thyrotoxicosis is associated with onycholysis and, when caused by Graves' disease, clubbing (thyroid achropachy). Koilonychia (spoon shaped nails) are seen in iron deficiency anaemias. Pitting, ribbing, and brittleness are often seen in severe illness and in malabsorption syndromes. Yellow nail syndrome is characterized by idiopathic pleural effusions, lymphoedema, chest infections, sinusitis, and yellow discolouration of the nails.

Answer 14

B Alopecia areata.

Scarring alopecia is permanent hair loss as a result of severe inflammation of the dermis with loss of hair follicles. The most common causes include:
- Lichen planus.
- Scleroderma.
- SLE.
- Tinea capitis.
- Staphylococcal folliculitis.
- Squamous cell and basal carcinoma.
- Scarring may also follow burns or exposure to erosive chemicals.

Alopecia areata causes localized nonscarring alpoecia. It is thought to be an autoimmune disease process with autosomal dominant inheritance. There is a higher incidence of this disorder in atopic individuals, stress, and Down's syndrome. It is characterized by the development of bald patches with no evidence of underlying skin disease or scarring. There may be associated pitting of the nails. In some cases there may be total hair loss. In patchy hair loss, the prognosis is good with 75% of patients recovering. More extensive hair loss is associated with a worse prognosis with an increased chance of recurrence.

Indicators of poor prognosis include:
- Onset in childhood.
- Atopy.
- Nail involvement.
- Loss of eyebrows.
- Loss of hair at the margins.

Trichotillomania is a disorder of psychiatric patients who pull their hair out. It is not scarring.

Question 15 Hypertrichosis is not a recognized feature of:

A Malnutrition.
B Porphyria.
C Treatment with penicillamine.
D Seborrhoeic dermatitis.
E Anorexia nervosa.

Question 16 The following is not associated with psoriasis:

A Ulcerative colitis.
B Sacroiliitis.
C Hyperuricaemia.
D Flattening of intestinal villi in erythroderma.
E Pustules in the epidermis.

Question 17 The following diseases may present with the following cutaneous lesions with the exception of:

A Rheumatoid arthritis and pyoderma gangrenosum.
B SLE and butterfly rash.
C Sjögren's syndrome and purpura.
D Rheumatic fever and erythema marginatum.
E Dermatomyositis and erythema nodosum.

Answer 15

D Seborrhoeic dermatitis.

Hypertrichosis describes excessive hair growth on any part of the body. It may be congenital or be secondary to systemic disease, or occurs as a result of side-effects of drugs. Gross malnutrition especially in children may result in generalized hypertrichosis. Congenital porphyria is a recognized cause, and hepatic porphyria induced by exposure to chemicals (hexachlorobenzene) is associated with marked hair growth on the face and extremities. Penicillamine induces an increased diameter and length of hairs on the trunk and thighs. Anorexia nervosa is associated with downy hypertrichosis on the face.

Tutorial

Other causes of hypertrichosis include:

- Dermatomyositis (associated with alopecia and generalized hypertrichosis).
- Hypothyroidism.
- Pregnancy.
- Drugs: Steroids, psoralens, diazoxide, minoxidil, cyclosporin A, streptomycin.
- Mercury poisoning (acrodynia).

Answer 16

A Ulcerative colitis.

Hyperuricaemia is a feature of severe psoriasis. Erythroderma is a very serious condition associated with marked debilitation. In severe systemic illness, flattening of the intestinal villi is common. Pustular psoraisis may be generalized and appear as numerous small, yellow, sterile pustules throughout the skin. Palmoplanter pustulosis is localized to the palms and soles and there is a strong association with smoking.

Psoriatic arthropathy (sero-negative) occurs in 10% of patients with cutaneous disease. This may take the form of:

- Ankylosing spondylitis associated with HLA B27, occurring in 5% of patients with psoriatic arthropathy.
- Asymmetrical oligoarthritis occurring in 70%.
- Rheumatoid type arthritis occurring in 15%.
- Asymmetrical arthritis involving the distal interphalangeal joints in 5%.
- Arthritis mutilans (5%) most commonly occurs in patients with severe cutaneous disease.

The arthritis may precede the onset of skin lesions and is usually independent of disease activity in the skin.

Ulcerative colitis is associated with erythema nodosum and pyoderma gangrenosum.

Answer 17

E Dermatomyositis and erythema nodosum.

Pyoderma gangrenosum occurs in rheumatoid arthritis. It is characterized by painful cutaneous ulceration with an undermined violaceous border, and most commonly occurs on the limbs (but the face and abdomen may be involved). Treatment is with high-dose steroids. Other skin manifestations of RA include:

- Livedo reticularis.
- Palpable purpura.
- Rash of JCA (salmon coloured morbilliform eruption on the trunk and proximal limbs).

Other causes of pyoderma gangrenosum include:

- IBD (ulcerative colitis, Crohn's).
- Paraproteinaemia.
- Myeloma.
- Wegener's granulomatosis.

The association of SLE and a butterfly rash is very well recognized affecting up to 80% of patients with this condition.

Sjögren's syndrome consists of a triad of xerostomia, keratoconjunctivitis sicca, and the sicca syndrome. Cutaneous manifestations include the development of palpable purpura. It is associated with anti-Ro (SS-a) and anti-La (SS-b) antibodies.

Erythema marginatum is a transient pink rash with raised edges affecting approximately 22% of patients with rheumatic fever. The erythematous lesions are seen most frequently on the trunk or around the mouth and classically coalesce to form crescent or ring shaped patches.

Morphea is a localized form of scleroderma. It can occur on the limbs and trunk as well as the face and scalp where it is referred to as *'en coup de sabre'*. It consists of indurated erythematous plaques with violaceous borders and hypopigmented sclerotic centres. Dermatomyositis is associated with a heliotrope rash affecting the eyelids and red scaling papules at the knuckles (Gottren's papules).

Question 18 The following is not true for erythema multiforme:

A Target lesions are characteristic.
B The palms and soles are frequently affected.
C Recurrent episodes are most commonly due to mycoplasma infection.
D May be a complication of penicillin treatment.
E Recovery may be complicated by arthropathy.

Question 19 The following is true for bullous pemphigoid:

A The condition is more common in men.
B Histology shows a split between the upper and lower portion of the epidermis.
C Circulating IgG or C3 antibodies to the basement membrane are found in 75% of patients.
D The mouth is often the only site affected.
E There is no association with underlying malignancy.

Answer 18

C Recurrent episodes are most commonly due to mycoplasma infection.

In erythema multiforme, the rash has a symmetrical distribution involving the face, limbs, trunk, palms, and soles. In severe cases, oral, ocular, and genital ulcers occur (Stevens–Johnson syndrome). It may be caused by infection with mycoplasma, although recurrent episodes are usually due to herpes simplex infection. Fifty percent of cases are idiopathic. Recovery may be complicated by persistent arthropathy.

Drugs implicated in causing erythema multiforme include:

- Penicillin.
- Sulphonamides.
- Salicylates.
- Cotrimoxazole.
- Phenothiazines.
- Chlorpropamide.
- Thiazide diuretics.
- Barbiturates.

Answer 19

C Circulating IgG or C3 antibodies to the basement membrane are found in 75% of patients.

Bullous pemphigoid is more common in women. It is an autoimmune disease which is more frequent in the elderly. It starts on the limbs and often spreads to the trunk. The mucous membranes are often involved with oral lesions occurring in 30%, but very rarely as the presenting feature.

Typically the lesions are large, tense blisters on an erythematous base.

Histology demonstrates a split at the basement membrane with infiltration of inflammatory cells. Direct immunofluorescence shows a linear band of IgG and C3 at the basement membrane. Serology demonstrates circulating IgG or C3 antibody to the basement membrane in 75% of patients. There is a vague association with underlying malignancy.

It is pemphigus that shows intra-epidermal separation on histology. Intra-epidermal deposition of IgG is seen throughout the dermis.

Clinically, the blisters have often ruptured leaving crusts. Any site can be affected, and in some patients the mouth is the only site affected.

5 Endocrinology

Question 1 Gynaecomastia:

A Is a recognized feature of hypothyroidism.
B When caused by cimetidine is as a result of inhibition of testosterone biosynthesis.
C Is associated with a karyotype of XXY.
D Occurs in peritoneal carcinoma.
E Occurs following prolonged periods of starvation.

Question 2 Recombinant human growth hormone treatment in an adult with growth hormone (GH) deficiency would not be recommended in the following situation:

A Severe GH deficiency.
B A perceived impairment to the quality of life.
C They are already receiving treatment for other pituitary deficiencies.
D Peak bone mass is achieved with normal GH response to ITT.
E Weight gain.

A 16-year-old male gives a 6-month history of generalized weakness. On examination, he has a short stature but normal secondary sexual development. The remainder of his examination is unremarkable and his blood pressure is 100/70 mmHg (13.3/9.3 kPa). Investigations: Hb 15.2 g/dl, WCC 5.9 × 10^9/l, Na^+ 134 mmol/l, K^+ 2.3 mmol/l, HCO_3^- 32 mmol/l, urea 5.3 mmol/l.

Question 3 The following would make the diagnosis of Bartter's syndrome likely:

A Co-existing pyelonephritis.
B Hyperreninaemia.
C Hypoplasia of the juxtaglomerular apparatus on biopsy.
D Response to bendrofluazide.
E Positive family history.

Answer 1

C Is associated with a karyotype of XXY.

Gynaecomastia:
- Is associated with a karyotype of XXY.
- Occurs in bronchogenic carcinoma.
- Occurs following refeeding after prolonged periods of starvation.

Gynaecomastia is a feature of thyrotoxicosis. Cimetidine inhibits the binding of testosterone to the androgen receptor. Spironolactone inhibits testosterone biosynthesis and hence causes gynaecomastia. Klinefelter's syndrome (XXY) is also a recognized cause. It may occur during the recovery period after prolonged starvation.

Tutorial

Causes of gynaecomastia:
Physiological (neonatal, pubertal, and senile):
- Drugs: oestrogens, aromatase androgens (testosterone ethanate or propionate), calcium channel blockers, ACE inhibitors, digoxin, amiodarone, spironolactone, phenothiazines, metoclopramide, TCAs, marijuana, cimetidine, omeprazole, isoniazid, metronidazole, busulphan, ketoconazole, and alcohol.
- Endocrine: hyperthyroidism, acromegaly, Cushing's syndrome, hyperprolactinaemia.
- Systemic disorders: chronic renal failure, hepatic cirrhosis.
- Tumours: leydig cell tumours may secrete oestrogens (or androgens which are aromatized to oestrogens). HCG stimulates oestrogen production, hence tumours secreting HCG are associated with gynaecomastia. Lung, kidney, and liver neoplasms may secrete HCG.
- Other: chest wall injury, herpes zoster, post thoracotomy.

Answer 2

E Weight gain.

Recombinant human growth hormone is recommended for the treatment of adults with growth hormone (GH) deficiency only if they fulfil all three of the following criteria:
- They have severe growth hormone deficiency as a peak response of <9 mU/l (3 ng/ml) during an insulin tolerance test.
- They have a perceived impairment of quality of life as demonstrated by a score of at least 11 in the disease specific questionnaire.
- They are already receiving treatment for any other pituitary hormone deficiencies.

Patients who develop GH deficiency in early adulthood, after linear growth is completed but before the age of 25 years should be given GH until adult peak bone mass has been achieved, provided they satisfy the criteria for severe GH deficiency. Weight gain may be a sign of GH deficiency but does not warrant treatment unless the above criteria are met.

Tutorial

Growth hormone is produced by the anterior pituitary gland and has a role in the regulation of protein, lipid, and carbohydrate metabolism as well as in increasing growth in children. Its secretion is intermittent and occurs predominantly during sleep. Secretion reaches maximal levels during adolescence and then declines with age by approximately 14% per decade.

Adult GH deficiency may be of adult onset or childhood onset and may occur as an isolated GH deficiency or as part of a multiple pituitary hormone deficiency. In adult onset GH, deficiency is commonly due to pituitary tumours or their treatment or due to cranial irradiation. Childhood onset is often idiopathic and may continue into adulthood. Iatrogenic GH deficiency may occur in both childhood or adulthood as a result of cranial irradiation or chemotherapy.

GH deficiency in adults may be associated with the following:
- Reduced quality of life.
- Reduced energy levels.
- Altered body composition (reduced lean mass and trunkal obesity).
- Osteopenia and osteoporosis.
- Dry skin (reduced sweating).
- Reduced muscle strength.
- Lipid abnormalities (elevated LDL).
- Increased levels of fibrinogen and plasminogen activator inhibitor.
- Impaired cardiac function.

Answer 3

B Hyperreninaemia.

The boy has a normal blood pressure, hypokalaemia, increased bicarbonate, and muscle weakness. Barrter's syndrome:

- Is characterized by hyperreninaemia.
- Is caused by impaired chloride reabsorbtion in the ascending loop of Henle.
- May be complicated by hypomagnesaemia.
- Is treated with NSAIDs.

The underlying abnormality in Bartter's syndrome is subnormal reabsorption of chloride in the thick ascending limb of the loop of Henle.

A reduction in chloride absorption results in a reduction in sodium absorption, and hence results in an increased sodium load in the distal nephron.

Due to an increase in the sodium being delivered to this site there is enhanced sodium–potassium exchange causing an increase in the distal tubular excretion of potassium. The overall effect of this is hypokalaemia which stimulates secretion of PGE2 from the renal cells and PGI2 from the vascular endothelium, causing chronic stimulation of renin secretion from the juxtaglomerular apparatus. The resultant effects are hyperreninaemia and high levels of circulating angiotensin II, and a moderate secondary hyperaldosteronism. Clinical features include kaluresis, hypokalaemic alkalosis, and normotension. Patients do not have oedema or evidence of loss of potassium and chloride from the gastrointestinal tract or symptoms due to laxatives or diuretics. Infrequently hypomagnesaemia occurs.

NSAIDs will inhibit cyclooxygenase and reduce PGE2 and PGI2 production, thereby reducing renin and aldosterone secretion.

The diagnosis of Bartter's syndrome can be supported by renal biopsy, where hyperplasia of the juxtaglomerular apparatus is characteristically seen. Pyelonephritis is a cause of hypokalaemia but does not occur as part of Bartter's syndrome.

Question 4 The following is not associated with insulin resistance:

A Sturge–Weber syndrome.
B Ataxia telangiectasia.
C Obesity.
D Cushing's syndrome.
E Acromegaly.

Question 5 The following is not true for phaeochromocytoma:

A Is associated with sustained hypertension in 50% of patients.
B Crisis may be precipitated by micturition.
C May occur in association with pituitary tumours in MEN type I.
D Patients may have *café-au-lait* spots.
E Medical treatment with alpha and beta blockade is the treatment of choice.

Question 6 The following is not true of neonatal hypothyroidism:

A May be caused by transfer of TRBAb across the placenta.
B Can occur in neonates born to mothers who have been iodine deficient during pregnancy.
C Is associated with jaundice.
D Is characterized by hypotonia.
E Microstomia is a recognized feature.

Question 7 A Barr body may not be found in buccal smears in:

A Turner's syndrome.
B A normal female.
C Klinefelter's syndrome.
D Sheehan's syndrome.
E An XY/XYY mosaic.

Answer 4

A Sturge–Weber syndrome.

Insulin resistance is characterized by normal or elevated levels of plasma glucose, in the presence of moderate to extreme elevations in serum insulin concentration.

Common causes of insulin resistance:
- Obesity.
- NIDDM.
- Polycystic ovaries.
- Pregnancy
- Acromegaly.
- Cushing's disease/syndrome.

Tutorial

Inherited insulin resistance may result from a variety of abnormalities:
- Pre-receptor, including genetic mutations that produce abnormal insulin molecules, or that result in the inability to cleave proinsulin into insulin and C peptide resulting in high circulating serum proinsulin levels.
- Receptor disorders result from a multitude of inactivating genetic mutations that affect the insulin receptor.
- Post-receptor disorders include loss of function mutations involving the insulin-receptor substrate 1 (IRS-1), glucose transporters, intracellular signalling proteins, and enzymes involved in intracellular glucose metabolism.

Insulin resistance is also a recognized feature of ataxia telangiectasia, an autosomal recessive condition consisting of marked telangiectasia of the nose, ears, conjunctiva, and skin creases, cerebellar ataxia, and impaired cell-mediated immunity. The underlying defect is believed to be due to a defect in DNA repair. Death occurs in the third decade as a result of infection or lymphoreticular malignancy.

Insulin resistance is not a feature of Sturge–Weber syndrome, which is associated with a port wine stain in trigeminal nerve distribution and a leptomeningeal angioma seen more commonly in the parieto-occipital region. Epilepsy is common with the manifestation of contralateral focal siezures. There may also be evidence for optic atrophy, glaucoma, exophthalmos, spacticity, and a low IQ. The condition is associated with cerebral calcification which is often seen on skull X-ray.

Answer 5

E Medical treatment with alpha and beta blockade is the treatment of choice.

Phaeochromocytoma:
- Is associated with sustained hypertension in 50% of patients.
- Crisis may be precipitated by micturition.
- Patients may have *café-au-lait* spots.

Phaeochromocytomas are rare, usually benign tumours arising from the chromaffin cells of the sympathoadrenal system. Ninety perent arise from the adrenal medulla, 8% from the organ of Zukerland and <2% from extraadrenal sites. Sustained hypertension occurs in 50% with paroxysmal hypertension in 40–50%.

Attacks may be precipitated by micturition with phaeochromocytomas arising in the bladder wall. They occur in association with medullary thyroid carcinoma and parathyroid adenoma or hyperplasia in MEN II. Neurofibromatosis, often with *café-au-lait* spots, occurs in 5% of patients with phaeochromocytoma. Treatment of choice is surgical removal.

Answer 6

E Microstomia is a recognized feature.

Neonatal hypothyroidism:
- May be caused by transfer of TRBAb across the placenta.
- Can occur in neonates born to mothers who have been iodine deficient during pregnancy.
- Is associated with jaundice.
- Is characterized by hypotonia.

A recognized cause of neonatal hypothyroidism is maternal transfer of thyroid receptor blocking antibody.

In geographic areas of iodine deficiency, maternal and therefore foetal iodine deficiency is the most common cause of congenital hypothyroidism. Excess iodine inadvertently taken by the mother or received through painting the cervix with iodine-containing antiseptics (as is done after antepartum rupture of amniotic membranes) or through painting the umbilical stump post-partum can produce transient neonatal hypothyroidism.

Clinical manifestations include: prolonged jaundice, lethargy, constipation, feeding problems, and cold to touch.

Signs include: skin mottling, umbilical hernia, jaundice, macroglossia, large frontanelles with wide sutures, distended abdomen, hoarse cry, hypotonia, dry skin, slow reflexes, and goitre.

Answer 7

A Turner's syndrome.

Barr bodies represent genetically inactive X chromosomes which appear as a distinctive mass of nuclear chromatin near the nuclear membrane. In keeping with the Lyon hypothesis, in cells with more than one X chromosome, there is random inactivation of all but one of the X chromosomes. A normal female hence has one Barr body, a female with Turner's syndrome has none, whilst a male with Klinefelter's syndrome (XXY) will also have a Barr body. A female with Sheehan's syndrome has an XX karyotype.

Another technique using stained smears of peripheral blood demonstrates a drumstick projection from the nucleus of polymorphonuclear leucocytes in females. The number of drumsticks is not related to the number of X chromosomes.

In males the F body (or Y chromatin) appears as a fluorescent spot on the interphase nuclei of cells stained with quinacrine. This test can also be performed on buccal smears.

Question 8 The following would make the diagnosis of De Queran's thyroiditis unlikely:

A A painless goitre.
B Transient hyper- or hypothyroidism.
C An elevated ESR.
D Infection by group A streptococcus.
E Circulating antithyroid antibodies.

Question 9 Amenorrhoea is not an expected finding in:

A Polycystic ovarian syndrome.
B Testicular feminization syndrome.
C Turner's syndrome.
D Pseudo-hypoparathyroidism.
E Sheehan's syndrome.

Question 10 The following is not true of thyrotoxicosis:

A Is caused most commonly by Graves' disease.
B Is a recognized occurrence in choriocarcinoma.
C May occur in association with testicular teratomas.
D Is not associated with a flat TRH response.
E Is associated with iodine therapy.

Question 11 The following is not true for leprechaunism:

A Is characterized by precocious puberty and ovarian hyperandrogenism.
B Inheritance is autosomal dominant.
C Is associated with dilated cardiomyopathy.
D Pseudohypertrophy of the muscles is a recognized feature.
E Acanthosis nigricans is a common finding.

Question 12 The following would be in keeping with a diagnosis of craniopharyngioma with the exception of:

A Tumours arising from Rathke's pouch.
B Peak incidence is in the second decade.
C Approximately 60% are cystic.
D Infrasellar calcification is a characteristic finding.
E May present with galactorrhoea.

Answer 8

A A painless goitre.

The specific agent responsible for subacute thyroiditis is not known, although viruses particularly Coxsackie, adenovirus, mumps, echovirus, influenza, and EBV have been implicated.

The goitre is classically painful and tender to touch. Pain is often preceded by myalgia, low-grade fever, and sore throat. Dysphagia is also common. Symptoms of hyperthyroidism such as tachycardia, weight loss, and nervousness occur in up to 50% of patients.

The ESR is usually elevated above 50 mm/hour and may be associated with a normochromic anaemia and mild leucocytosis. T4 and T3 are elevated, as are anti-microsomal and antithyroglobulin antibodies (probably due to release of thyroglobulin into the circulation caused by damage to the gland, rather than an auto-immune response).

Answer 9

A Polycystic ovarian syndrome.

Primary amenorrhoea can be the presenting complaint in patients with testicular feminization, who do not have a uterus, and in Turner's syndrome where there is gonadal dysgenesis. In pseudo-hypoparathyroidism there is resistance to PTH, a cAMP-mediated hormone. Resistance to other cAMP-mediated hormones especially LH and FSH can occur resulting in amenorrhoea, although this is not to be expected in the majority of cases. Polycystic ovarian syndrome is associated with oligomenorrhoea. Sheehan's syndrome is a recognized cause of secondary amenorrhoea due to hypopituitarism.

Answer 10

D Is not associated with a flat TRH response.

Thyrotoxicosis:
- Is caused most commonly by Graves' disease.
- Is a recognized occurrence in choriocarcinoma.
- May occur in association with testicular teratomas.
- Is always associated with a flat TRH response.
- Is associated with iodine therapy.

Thyrotoxicosis is associated with all the examples. The commonest cause of hyperthyroidism is Graves's disease. Other causes consist of solitary toxic adenoma, toxic nodular goitre, acute thyroiditis (viral, autoimmune, and post radiation), thyrotoxicosis facticia, exogenous iodine, metastatic differentiated thyroid carcinomas, TSH-producing tumours (pituitary and ovarian), and HCG-producing tumours (testicular and choriocarcinoma).

Tutorial

TRH test
Hypothyroid patients have a high basal TSH level and demonstrate an exaggerated rise in response to TRH. Thyrotoxic patients have a suppressed TSH with a minimal rise in response to TRH. This is often referred to as a flat response.

A flat TRH response is seen in:
- Thyrotoxicosis.
- Solitary autonomous nodules.
- Grave's eye disease.
- Excessive thyroxine replacement.

Answer 11

B Inheritance is autosomal dominant.

Leprechaunism shows autosomal recessive inheritance. The underlying abnormality is as a result of insulin receptor mutations. Features consist of intrauterine and postnatal growth retardation, dysmorphic facies, lipo-dystrophy, muscle wasting, acanthosis nigricans, ovarian hyperandrogenism, precocious puberty, hypertrophic cardiomyopathy, and early death.

Answer 12

D Infrasellar calcification is a characteristic finding.

The following would be in keeping with a diagnosis of craniopharyngioma:
- Tumours arising from Rathke's pouch.
- Peak incidence is in the second decade.
- Approximately 60% are cystic.
- May present with galactorrhoea.

Craniopharyngiomas are usually calcified, often cystic and lie above the pituitary fossa. For this reason they are often referred to as suprasellar cysts. Skull X-rays are abnormal in 50% of patients. The commonest clinical presentations are headaches, visual field defects, growth failure (50% occur before age 20 years), and features of hypopituitarism (hyperprolactinaemia, stalk damage with DI). This hyperprolactinaemia may manifest itself with infertility, galactorrhoea, and hypogonadism.

Some patients present with hypothalamic syndromes, i.e. disturbance of sleep, appetite, and temperature regulation. There is a good response to treatment with surgery or radiotherapy.

Question 13 The following is not true for congenital adrenal hyperplasia:

A Is associated with increased serum levels of ACTH.
B Deficiency of 17-hydroxylase activity is the commonest cause.
C 21-hydroxylase deficiency is associated with precocious puberty.
D 11-β-hydroxylase deficiency is associated with hypertension and hypokalaemia.
E Prenatal diagnosis is possible in the first trimester using chorionic villous cells for HLA typing and molecular genetic studies.

Question 14 Hypoglycaemia is not a recognized feature of:

A Hypothyroidism.
B Addison's disease.
C Septicaemia.
D Large mesenchymal tumours.
E Phaeochromocytoma.

Question 15 The following is a recognized feature of anorexia nervosa:

A Serum growth hormone is reduced.
B Plasma gonadotrophins are high.
C The ESR is high.
D Patients often complain of a reduced appetite.
E May be complicated by recurrent infections and osteoporosis.

Question 16 A predictor of better outcome in patients with anorexia nervosa is:

A Low weight at diagnosis.
B Younger age of onset.
C Longer duration of illness.
D Disturbed family relationships.
E Repeated hospital admissions.

Answer 13

B Deficiency of 17-hydroxylase activity is the commonest cause.

CAH :

- Is associated with increased serum levels of ACTH.
- 21-hydroxylase deficiency is associated with precocious puberty.
- 11-β-hydroxylase deficiency is associated with hypertension and hypokalaemia.
- Prenatal diagnosis is possible in the first trimester using chorionic villous cells for HLA typing and molecular genetic studies.

Congenital adrenal hyperplasia is a family of autosomal recessive disorders of adrenal steroidogenesis in which there is deficient activity of one of the enzymes necessary for cortisol synthesis. As a result ACTH secretion is stimulated via negative feedback, causing adrenal hyperplasia and overproduction of the adrenal steroids. Both ACTH and steroid production precede the step that is deficient and so do not require the disordered enzyme.

21-hydroxylase deficiency is the commonest cause accounting for up to 90% of cases. Treatment is based on replacing cortisol to prevent further excessive ACTH secretion. In many cases there is significant virilization which will require surgical correction. Prenatal diagnosis is now possible in the first trimester of pregnancy.

11-β-hydroxylase deficiency is associated with hypertension and hypokalaemia.

Answer 14

E Phaeochromocytoma.

Hypoglycaemia can be caused by Addison's disease and septicaemia. Mesenchymal tumours may secrete insulin-like growth factor IGF-II which causes hypoglycaemia. Hypothyroidism is a recognized cause of hypoglycaemia, particularly in neonates. Phaeochromocytoma and thyrotoxicosis are associated with impaired glucose tolerance and glycosuria.

Tutorial

Other nonbeta cell tumours associated with hypoglycaemia include:

- Hepatocellular carcinoma (25%).
- Adrenal carcinomas (5–10%).
- Gastrointestinal tumours (5–10%).
- Lymphomas (5–10%).
- Carcinoma of kidney.
- Carcinoma of lung.
- Anaplastic carcinomas.
- Carcinoid.

Answer 15

E May be complicated by recurrent infections and osteoporosis.

In anorexia nervosa plasma gonadotrophins are low. Long term malnutrition is associated with risk of sepsis and osteoporosis. Serum growth hormone may be elevated in anorexia due to effects of starvation and excercise. The ESR is low. Patients often lie about eating and deny hunger.

Answer 16

B Younger age of onset.

The following are associated with a poor predicted outcome in anorexia nervosa:

- Low weight at diagnosis.
- Older age of onset.
- Longer duration of illness.
- Disturbed family relationships.
- Repeated hospital admissions.

Question 17 Cutaneous manifestations of diabetes mellitus do not include:

A Necrobiosis lipoidicum.
B Erythema nodosum.
C Vitiligo.
D Granuloma annulare.
E Acanthosis ngricans.

Question 18 The following is true for treatment with oral hypoglycaemics:

A Are the treatments of choice in hyperosmolar nonketotic states.
B Are safe in pregnancy.
C Hypoglycaemia is rarely caused by metformin.
D Treatment with metformin may be complicated by constipation.
E Chlorpropamide is used in preference to tolbutamide in the elderly.

Question 19 Complications of acute diabetic ketoacidosis and its treatment include:

A Gastrointestinal haemorrhage.
B Pneumothorax.
C Cerebral oedema.
D Cardiac arrest.
E Myopathy.

Question 20 Features of acromegaly do not include:

A Osteoporosis.
B Sleep apnoea.
C Increased risks of colonic carcinoma.
D Carpal tunnel syndrome.
E Hypoglycaemia.

Question 21 A short stature is not characteristic of:

A Turner's syndrome.
B Pseudohypoparathyroidism.
C Congenital adrenal hyperplasia.
D Down's syndrome.
E Obesity.

Question 22 The following is true with reference to calcitonin:

A Is a steroid hormone.
B Is produced in the parafollicular C-cells of the thyroid gland.
C Increases bone resorption by stimulating osteoblastic activity.
D Is a major tumour marker for papillary carcinoma of the thyroid.
E Promotes an increase in serum phosphate.

Answer 17

B Erythema nodosum.

In diabetes mellitus necrobiosis and granuloma annulare are recognized cutaneous complications of diabetes. Vitiligo may occur in type 1 as part of an autoimmune polyglandular disorder. Erythema nodosum is not a feature of diabetes mellitus.

Answer 18

C Hypoglycaemia is rarely caused by metformin.

Metformin very rarely causes hypoglycaemia. Insulin is the treatment of choice in HONC. All pregnant women should be converted to insulin unless (in the rare circumstance) their glycaemic control is meticulous on diet alone. Chlorpropamide is long acting, and hence should be avoided in the elderly.

Answer 19

E Myopathy.

All of the examples except myopathy can be complications of acute diabetic ketoacidosis and its treatment. Gastrointestinal haemorrhage may occur as a result of stress ulceration. Pneumothorax can occur on inserting a central line and cerebral oedema from overzealous fluid replacement. Cardiac arrest can occur as a result of electrolyte imbalance, particularly potassium, and hypokalaemia may cause muscle weakness, but not myopathy.

Answer 20

E Hypoglycaemia.

In patients with acromegaly sleep apnoea is common. Colonic polyps are well documented, and their malignant transformation calls for polypectomy and recurrent colonoscopies when diagnosed. Increased serum IGF-I reflects a state of active acromegaly. Acromegaly is frequently complicated by osteoarthritis. Carpal tunnel syndrome, particularly bilateral in the nonpregnant patient, should alert one to look for other features of acromegaly. Patients with acromegaly are insulin resistant and hyperglycaemia is a common feature.

Answer 21

E Obesity.

Causes of short stature:

- Familial.
- Nutritional: starvation, malabsorption, e.g. coeliac and Crohn's disease.
- Genetic defects: Turner's and Down's syndrome.
- Endocrine: hypothyroidism, hypopituitarism, CAH, sexual precocity, Cushing's disease.
- Skeletal disorders: rickets, achondroplasia.
- Systemic disease: renal failure, cyanotic congenital heart disease, TB, anaemia.

Tutorial

Causes of tall stature:

- GH-secreting tumours.
- Cerebral gigantism (Soto's syndrome: tall stature, prominent forehead, high arched palate, antimongoloid slant of palpebral fissures, mental retardation, and advanced bone age. Endocrine tests are normal.)
- Marfan's syndrome, homocystinuria.
- Klinefelter's syndrome.
- Untreated prepubertal CAH.
- Precocious secretion of oestrogens and androgens.
- Obesity.

Answer 22

B Is produced in the parafollicular C-cells of the thyroid gland.

Calcitonin is a 32-amino acid polypeptide. It is produced in the parafollicular C-cells in the thyroid and is a marker for medullary carcinoma of the thyroid. It reduces bone resorption by inhibiting osteoclast activity and augments osteoblastic activity, promoting bone formation. It acts on the kidney to reduce calcium absorption and causes a net reduction in serum calcium and phosphate.

Calcitonin is decreased in the short term by a fall in the serum calcium and is maintained in the long term by oestrogen and testosterone, which is important in the prevention of osteoporosis. It can be modulated by several of the gastrointestinal hormones including gastrin.

Tutorial

Causes of increased serum calcitonin:
- Physiological: pregnancy, OCP, breast feeding, infancy.
- Malignancy: medullary carcinoma of the thyroid, phaeochromocytoma, carcinoid, oat cell carcinoma of the bronchus.
- Myeloid leukaemia.
- Hyperparathyroidism.
- Megaloblastic anaemia.
- Chronic lung disease.

Causes of reduced serum calcitonin:
- Old age.
- Male sex.
- Hypogonadism.

Question 23 The following is true for congenital adrenal hyperplasia:

A Inheritance is sex-linked.
B Serum ACTH levels are suppressed.
C 21-hydroxylase deficiency is the most common type.
D Salt losing crisis is unusual in neonates.
E Serum androstenedione levels are characteristically low.

Question 24 Polcystic ovarian syndrome is associated with:

A A positive family history.
B Raised serum levels of dehydroepiandrosterone sulphate (DHEAS).
C A high FSH to LH ratio.
D A high steroid hormone-binding globulin.
E Characteristically presents with amenorrhoea.

Question 25 Cranial diabetes insipidus is not characterized by:

A A urine volume of >3 litres/day.
B A urine osmolality of <300 mOsm/kg.
C Raised plasma osmolality.
D Increasing circulating levels of vasopressin.
E In cranial diabetes insipidus the urine osmolality remains below that of the serum during water deprivation.

Answer 23

C 21-hydroxylase deficiency is the most common type.

Congenital adrenal hyperplasia is a family of autosomal recessive disorders of adrenal steroidogenesis in which there is deficient activity of one of the enzymes necessary for cortisol synthesis. 21-hydroxylase deficiency is the most common type, accounting for 90% of cases. Inadequate 21-hydroxylation of progesterone results in aldosterone deficiency, and salt wasting crisis may occur in 75% of affected infants.

ACTH levels are high as a result of negative feedback, causing adrenal hyperplasia and overproduction of steroids. ACTH and steroid production precede the step that is deficient and so do not require the disordered enzyme. There is excessive adrenal androgen production and this is mainly in the form of androstenedione. This is responsible for the virilization which is the hallmark of the disorder. Serum 17-hydroxyprogesterone is elevated, as is the urine pregnanetriol. Treatment is with steroids which act by suppressing ACTH.

Clinical features include:
- Ambiguous genitalia at birth.
- Virilization in the female and precocious puberty in the male.
- Rapid growth but eventual short stature.

Answer 24

A A positive family history.

In polycystic ovarian syndrome there is a positive family history. The enlarged ovaries secrete excess androgens from theca and stromal cell hyperplasia.

Endocrine changes:
- Increased LH to FSH ratio.
- DHEAS is a unique adrenal androgen. Urinary 17-ketosteroids are normal.
- The steroid hormone-binding globulin is low.
- Oestradiol levels are low.
- The prolactin and testosterone are slightly raised.

Physical signs include:
- Obesity.
- Hirsutism.
- Oligomenorrhoea.
- Acne.
- Mild virilization occurs in severe cases.
- Infertility.

Ultrasound shows bilateral polycystic ovaries. Infertility is treated with clomiphene.

Answer 25

D Increasing circulating levels of vasopressin.

Diabetes insipidus is characterized by hypotonic polyuria. Classic laboratory findings include:
- Large urinary volume of >3 litres/day.
- Urine osmolality of <200–300 mOsm/kg.
- Slightly elevated plasma osmolality.
- In cranial DI the serum ADH is low despite slightly elevated serum osmolality.
- In nephrogenic DI the levels of ADH are normal or high.

Features of cranial diabetes insipidis include high or high-normal plasma osmolality with low urine osmolality, with a resultant high or high-normal sodium. There is failure of urinary concentration following fluid deprivation, and the restoration of urinary concentration with vasopressin.

6 Gastroenterology

Question 1 The following is not true of Hirchsprung's disease:

A May present at birth with intestinal obstruction.
B Is due to an aquired absence of the myenteric nerves in the Auerbach's plexus.
C Can be diagnosed by full thickness rectal biopsy.
D Pressure studies show failure of relaxation of the internal sphincter.
E Barium enema demonstrates a narrowed aganglionic segment.

Question 2 The following is not true for oesophageal carcinoma:

A Occurs more frequently in patients with coeliac disease.
B Is associated with recurrent gastro-oesophageal reflux.
C Tumours are most frequently squamous in histology.
D Risks of malignant change are reduced on treatment of achalasia.
E Alcoholism is a recognized predisposing factor.

Question 3 The following is not an aetiological factor in acute pancreatitis:

A Alcoholic binges.
B Secondary hyperparathyroidism.
C Hypothermia.
D Thiazide diuretics.
E Polyarteritis nodosa.

Question 4 The following is true for coeliac disease:

A Is more common in males.
B Is associated with HLA B27.
C Is characterized by increased intestinal lactase activity.
D Proximal small bowel is less affected than the ileum.
E Is associated with an increased incidence of atopy.

Answer 1

B Is due to an aquired absence of the myenteric nerves in the Auerbach's plexus.

Hirschsprung's disease often presents in the first week of life with intestinal obstruction. It may, however, present later in the neonatal period with chronic constipation, anorexia, failure to thrive, and growth retardation. It is a congenital disorder in which there is a localized absence of the myenteric nerves in Auerbach's plexus. Failure of relaxation of the internal sphincter on pressure studies is diagnostic of Hirschsprung's disease. Barium enema demonstrates a narrowed aganglionic segment.

A full thickness rectal biopsy is necessary to demonstrate the absence of ganglionic cells. There is a tenfold increase of Hirchsprung's disease in Down's syndrome.

Tutorial

In 70% of cases, the rectosigmoid is involved, in 20% the colon is involved proximal to the sigmoid, and in 10% the aganglionosis extends proximally to the small intestine. It is not associated with a high incidence of prematurity and the majority of babies have a birth weight appropriate for their gestational age. This is in marked contrast to other congenital GI tract malformations.

Answer 2

D Risks of malignant change are reduced on treatment of achalasia.

Increased risk of oesophageal carcinoma is associated with the following conditions: achalasia of the cardia, Barret's oesophagus (which is due to acid reflux), Plummer–Vinson syndrome (iron deficiency anaemia with pharyngeal web), familial tylosis, and coeliac disease. Coeliac is more frequently associated with small bowel lymphoma. Squamous carcinomas account for most oesophageal malignancies, except for in the lower third where adenocarcinomas are more common and may arise from the fundus of the stomach. Fifty percent of malignancies occur in the middle, and 25% in the lower third of the oesophagus.

There is an increased prevalence in China, Africa, and the Caspian region of Iran. In the UK it accounts for 2.5% of all malignancies, and is more common in smokers (adenocarcinoma and squamous carcinoma) and heavy alcohol drinkers (squamous carcinoma). Other factors associated with increased risk include mouldy foods and diets deficient in molybdenum, vitamins A, C and riboflavin. Caustic strictures are also associated with a higher risk of oesophageal malignancy.

More than 90% of patients present with progressive dysphagia. Barium swallow is the initial investigation of choice, followed by oesophagoscopy and biopsy. Five-year survival is 2%.

Answer 3

B Secondary hyperparathyroidism.

Causes of acute pacreatitis include gall stones (40%), alcoholic binges, drugs, e.g thiazides, steroids, oestrogens, valproate, sulphonamides, tetracyclines, and azathioprine, viral infections, e.g. mumps, Coxsackie B, hypercalcaemia, and hypothermia. In addition, causes of acute pancreatitis can be iatrogenic, e.g. post surgical or post ERCP, hyperlipidaemia especially Fredrickson's type I and V, and pancreatic tumours. Ischaemia as a result of hypotension or vasculitis such as PAN may also result in acute pancreatitis. In some 40% of cases no cause can be found and these may be referred to as idiopathic.

Other causes include scorpion bite, pregnancy, and hereditary causes. In secondary hyperparathyroidism the calcium is normal.

Answer 4

E Is associated with an increased incidence of atopy.

Tutorial

Coeliac disease shows a female preponderance. It can present at any age, becoming apparent in infancy on weaning with gluten-containing foods. In adults the peak incidence is in the third to fourth decade. There is an increased incidence in families with 10–15% of siblings affected. Eighty percent have HLA B8 DR3 (which occurs in 25% of the normal population). The B8 component is as a result of linkage disequilibrium.

Ninety percent of patients have class 2 antigen DQW2. In the bowel intestinal lactase activity and nutrient absorption are reduced and permeability is increased. Mucosa of the proximal bowel is predominantly affected, with reduction in severity towards the ileum where the gluten has been digested to nontoxic fragments.

Diagnosis is made on duodenal biopsy as opposed to ileum. There is an increased incidence of atopy and other autoimmune disease, especially thyroiditis, IDDM, chronic liver disease, IBD, and fibrosing and allergic alveolitis. Antigliadin and antireticulin antibodies can be demonstrated in the serum.

Complications

Coeliac disease must be regarded as a premalignant condition as small bowel lymphoma may supervene usually at or beyond middle age. Symptoms suggestive of lymphoma include deterioration of health, abdominal discomfort and diarrhoea despite keeping to a gluten free diet, gastrointestinal bleeding, or skin rashes. Signs include anaemia, lymphadenopathy, clubbing, abdominal distension, and hepatomegaly.

Obstruction or perforation of the small intestine may occur. Carcinoma of the oesophagus or jejunum have also been reported. Atrophy of the spleen occurs in some adult patients with coeliac disease.

Question 5 Malabsorption is not a recognized feature of:

A Whipple's disease.
B Acarbose treatment.
C Giardiasis.
D Methotrexate therapy.
E Crohn's disease.

Question 6 The following is not true of ulcerative colitis:

A May be complicated by carcinoma of the oesophagus.
B Is associated with an increased incidence of deep vein thrombosis.
C May be complicated by erythema multiforme.
D Loss of haustral pattern is often apparent on barium enema.
E Rectal mucosa is always involved.

Question 7 The following is true of medical treatment of ulcerative colitis:

A Is unlikely to affect fertility in patients on sulphasalazine.
B Hypoglycaemia may be a feature during treatment of an acute exacerbation.
C Caution should be shown in slow acetylators.
D May be complicated by polycythaemia.
E Lung fibrosis is not a a recognized side-effect of sulphasalazine.

Answer 5

E Crohn's disease.

Whipple's disease, Crohn's disease and giardiasis are well recognized causes of malabsorption. Acarbose acts by impaired carbohydrate absorption.

Sulphasalazine and phenytoin commonly cause folate malabsorption. Many other drugs can also cause malabsorption, though this is of little clinical significance (see Tutorial).

Tutorial

Causes of malabsorption

Mucosal (diagnosed by intestinal biopsy):
- Coeliac disease.
- Dermatitis herpetiformis.
- Cow's milk sensitivity in infants.
- Whipple's disease.
- Intestinal lymphangiectasia.
- Abetalipoproteinaemia.

Structural (usually diagnosed with small bowel radiography):
- Gastric surgery.
- Crohn's disease.
- Ulcerative colitis.
- Intestinal resection.
- Blind loops, intestinal fistulae, diverticulae.
- Small intestine lymphoma or malignancy.
- Pancreatic atrophy.

Infective:
- Acute enteritis.
- Travellers' diarrhoea.
- Intestinal tuberculosis.
- Giardiasis.
- Whipple's disease (also mucosal).

Defective luminal digestion:
- Chronic pancreatitis.
- Carcinoma of the pancreas.
- Cystic fibrosis.
- Zollinger–Ellison syndrome.
- Parenchymal liver disease.
- Biliary obstruction.
- Terminal ileum disease.

Disease outside the GI tract:
- Hyper/hypothyroidism.
- Addison's disease.
- Hyper/hypoparathyroidism.
- Carcinoid syndrome.

Drugs

Drugs that may cause malabsorption of little clinical significance:
- Methotrexate.
- Colchicine.
- Metformin.
- Laxatives.
- Salicylates.
- Neomycin.

Drugs that may cause diarrhoea:
- Antibiotics.*
- Laxatives.
- Beta-blockers.**
- Magnesium-containing antacids.
- Olsalazine.
- Iron.
- Mefenamic acid.
- Biguanides.
- Misoprostol.***

* Due to disruption of colonic flora which may result in unnecessary infection by *Clostridium difficile.*

** Beta-blockers antagonize adrenergic antiperistaltic action.

*** Misoprostol stimulates intestinal motility and secretion.

Drugs that may cause constipation:
- Opiates.
- Antimuscarinics (tricyclic antidepressants, atropine, phenothiazines).
- Aluminium-containing antacids.
- Sucralfate.
- Iron.

Answer 6

A May be complicated by carcinoma of the oesophagus.

Recognized complications of ulcerative colitis include:
- May be complicated by carcinoma of the bile duct.
- Is associated with an increased incidence of deep vein thrombosis.
- May be complicated by erythema multiforme.

- Loss of haustral pattern is often apparent on barium enema.
- Rectal mucosa is always involved.

Liver complications of ulcerative colitis include fatty infiltration, chronic active hepatitis, and pericholangitis (which are common), and sclerosing cholangitis, ascending cholangitis, and carcinoma of the bile duct, which are less common. Five percent of cases are complicated by DVT.

Skin complications include erythema nodosum (2%), pyoderma gangrenosum, leg ulcers (2%), and, rarely, erythema multiforme. Barium enema may show loss of haustral pattern with shortening of the bowel to give a smooth tube hosepipe appearance. The rectal mucosa is virtually always abnormal. Other complications include iritis, episcleritis (5%), stomatitis (15%), arthropathy (15%, usually affecting large joints, symmetrical and non-deforming), apthous ulcers, clubbing, and secondary amyloidosis.

Answer 7

C Caution should be shown in slow acetylators.

Recognized complications of medical treatment of ulcerative colitis include:

- May be complicated by fertility in patients on sulphasalazine.
- Hypoglycaemia may be a feature during treatment of an acute exacerbation.
- Caution should be shown in slow acetylators.
- May be complicated by polycythaemia.
- Lung fibrosis is not a a recognized side-effect of sulphasalazine.

Side-effects of sulphasalazine include reduced sperm count, agranulocytosis, lung fibrosis, nausea, vomiting, epigastric discomfort, rashes, headaches, neutropenia, thrombocytopenia, Stevens–Johnson syndrome, and SLE-like syndrome. Caution must be shown in slow acetylators. High-dose steroids used in acute exacerbations may produce diabetogenic effects, hence cause symptomatic hyperglycaemia.

Question 8 The following is not true for Whipple's disease:

A Is caused by *Tropheryma whippeli.*
B Diagnosis can be confirmed by gastric biopsy.
C Patients often have skin pigmentation.
D Lymphadenopathy is characteristic.
E Oculomasticatory myerrhythmia is diagnostic.

Question 9 The following is not true with reference to proctitis:

A When caused by chlamydia, may be associated with haemorrhage.
B Is a recognized complication of bacillary dysentery.
C Ischaemia is a common cause.
D Is a feature of gay bowel syndrome.
E May occur in association with a positive pathogen test.

Question 10 The following is true with reference to liver biopsy:

A Is safe in the presence of ascites.
B Is the investigation of choice when a liver abscess is suspected.
C May be complicated by septic shock.
D Haemangioma of the liver is a relative contraindication.
E Mortality is >2%.

Answer 8

B Diagnosis can be confirmed by gastric biopsy.

Whipple's disease is caused by Gram-negative actinomycete *Tropheryma whippeli*. Common features of infection include malabsorption which is almost always present, skin pigmentation, peripheral lymphadenopathy, arthralgia, abdominal pain, diarrhoea, progressive weight loss, and low-grade fever. Most patients have episodes of a migratory polyarthritis affecting the large joints and remitting without any deformity. Less common features include neurological manifestations such as confusion, memory loss, focal cranial nerve lesions, and ophthalmoplegia.

Oculomasticatory myerrhythmia is diagnostic. Duodenal biopsy shows dilated lacteals in the bowel wall with macrophages containing cytoplasmic granules which are PAS-positive in the lamina propria. Malabsorption results in steatorrhoea, anaemia, and hypoalbuminaemia. Treatment is with trimethoprim and sulphamethoxazole for 12 months.

Answer 9

C Ischaemia is a common cause.

Proctitis is associated with stinging rectal pain and pus. Bacillary dysentery (shigella) is a well-recognized cause, as is the protozoan *Entamoeba histolytica*, which can also be transmitted by anal intercourse and is otherwise referred to as gay bowel syndrome. The differential diagnosis for proctitis is large, and can be divided into infective, inflammatory, and radiation. Infective causes include *Chlamydia trachomatis*, which is transmitted in this case by anal intercourse and causes a haemorrhagic proctocolitis with regional lymphadenitis, which may become suppurative as in lymphogranuloma venerum. Herpes simplex, HIV, and gonorrhoea can also cause a proctitis, and inflammatory bowel disease is a very common cause. Ischaemic proctitis is rare due to the good collateral supply via the iliac arteries. Behçet's disease is associated with a positive pathogen test and may present with proctitis, although oral and genital ulcers are the more common cause of presentation.

Answer 10

C May be complicated by septic shock.

Relative contraindications for percutaneous liver biopsy include ascites, jaundice, platelet count <80, PT >3 seconds above control (which is associated with an increased risk of haemorrhage), and respiratory disease which may prevent the patient from controlling his own respiration and increases the risk of a capsular tear. Bacteraemia is known to occur in 15% of patients; the organisms are most often Gram-negative, and septic shock is a recognized complication. Liver biopsy is absolutely contraindicated in haemangioma of the liver and in suspected liver abscess, where CT guided drainage is more favourable.

Table: Liver biopsy appearances

Infections

Acute viral hepatitis (A, B, C). Panlobular necrosis, ballooning and acidophil degeneration; bridging necrosis is associated with a poor prognosis.

Chronic hepatitis (A,B,C). Chronic persistent hepatitis: normal architecture, mononuclear mainly lymphocyte infiltration in portal tracts which may be expanded by fibrous spurs.

Herpes simplex. Haemorrhagic necrosis; intranuclear inclusions.

Cytomegalovirus. Like viral hepatitis with CMV inclusions in >20%.

Rickettsial (Q fever). Focal necrosis with granulomas and a mononuclear infiltrate.

Leprosy and tuberculosis. Epithelioid granulomas with acid-fast bacilli.

Brucellosis. Microgranulomas, positive culture is rare.

Syphilis. Secondary: nonspecific changes with hepatitis and spirochaetes.
Late: gummatous, resembling tumours.

Leptospirosis. Nonspecific focal necrosis and cholestasis.

Neoplasms
Hepatocellular carcinoma. Plates of cells resembling hepatocytes.

Metastases. Varies with primary site, usually adenocarcinoma or anaplastic.

Lymphoma or leukaemia. Usually not diagnostic.

Question 11 The following is not true of fatty infiltration of the liver:

A Is a feature of Wilson's disease.
B Commonly occurs in kwashiorkor.
C May be segmental, lobar, or spotty.
D Is dark on ultrasound.
E Occurs in patients on TPN.

Question 12 The following is true of primary biliary cirrhosis:

A Is associated with copper deposition in the liver.
B Is associated with polyarteritis nodosa.
C IgM levels are low.
D Is associated with prolonged bile duct obstruction.
E High levels of antimitochondrial muscle antibody is associated with a worse prognosis.

Question 13 The conjugation of bilirubin:

A Is catalysed by glucuronyl transferase.
B Takes place in the kupffer cells of the liver.
C Is aided by sulphonamides.
D Is partly inhibited by phenobarbitone.
E Is efficient in the premature infant.

Question 14 The following is true of amoebic liver abscess:

A Develops most commonly after a recent bout of colitis.
B Aspiration yields a characteristic straw coloured fluid.
C Serology may be negative.
D Chest X-ray often shows elevation of the left hemidiaphragm.
E Abscesses occur more frequently in the right lobe of the liver.

Answer 11

D Is dark on ultrasound.

Fatty infiltration of the liver can occur in a number of conditions including obesity, pregnancy, alcoholism, diabetes mellitus, inflammatory bowel disease, starvation (hence kwashiorkor), early stages of chronic liver disorders, e.g. Wilson's disease, and conditions associated with general debility and malnutrition such as TB and cystic fibrosis. Patients on TPN may have chronic illness and be malnourished, and frequently have mildly elevated ALT and AST. There is no liver cell damage and fatty change itself is not a precirrhotic condition. In very severe fatty change, e.g. malnutrition and alcoholism, marked changes in all LFTs can occur.

Tutorial

Ultrasound of the liver is safe, cheap, and accurate in experienced hands.

Fat is bright on ultrasound and the pattern can vary, being uniform, segmental, or spotty. Abscesses appear as black transonic areas surrounded by high intensity areas. Cysts have black transonic areas surrounded by a thin echogenic rim.

Neoplasia produces areas of discontinuity in areas of homogenous liver.

Metastases produce an amplitude that is less than that of the surrounding liver but colonic metastases produce high intensity echoes. Cirrhosis produces a higher amplitude of echoes than does the normal liver and a large portal vein may be demonstrated. In heart failure, the hepatic veins may be dilated.

Answer 12

A Is associated with copper deposition in the liver.

Primary biliary cirrhosis is associated with cholestasis and hence copper deposition in the liver, which is of a far lesser degree than in Wilson's disease.

Tutorial

The exact aetiology of PBC is unknown, but immunological mechanisms play a significant role and may account for both an increased incidence of connective tissue diseases, in particular scleroderma, rheumatoid arthritis, Sjögren's syndrome, and also conditions such as renal tubular acidosis, membranous glomerular nephritis, pancreatic atrophy, and the sicca complex which occurs in up to 70% of patients.

Mitochondrial antibodies are seen in >95% of patients but are not specific for this condition, occurring also in HbsAG-negative chronic active hepatitis. The presence of a high titre of this antibody is not related to the severity of the disease. Other antibodies occurring which are also specific are antinuclear factor and smooth muscle antibodies. Serum IgM may also be high. PBC is a disease of middle-aged women (male to female ratio 1:8). The earliest symptom is pruritus which precedes jaundice and hepatomegaly by 2–3 years. Liver biopsy shows portal tract inflammation, bile duct proliferation, centrizonal cholestasis, and granulomas. Secondary biliary cirrhosis occurs as a result of prolonged bile duct obstruction.

Answer 13

A Is catalysed by glucuronyl transferase.

Bilirubin is conjugated in the endoplasmic recticulum of the hepatocytes. The reaction is catalysed by enzyme glucuronyl transferase and is deficient in the premature infant. Eighty-five percent of bilirubin is formed from red cell breakdown, which occurs in the kupffer cells of the liver and in the rectoendothelial system. The remainder is formed from myoglobin, cytochromes, and catalases. 250–300 mg of bilirubin is produced daily and the unconjugated form is transported bound to albumin. In the liver, transporter proteins Y and Z carry it to the ER. Certain drugs, e.g. sulphonamides and salicylates decrease protein binding of unconjugated bilirubin.

Answer 14

E Abscesses occur more frequently in the right lobe of the liver.

The causative organism of amoebic liver abscess is *Entamoeba histolytica*, and the presentation is usually with a high swinging pyrexia, malaise, anorexia, and weight loss. Aspiration yields an anchovy sauce. On examination there is tender hepatomegaly and dullness at the right base of the chest. Serology, e.g. haemagglutination inhibition, amoebic complement fixation, and ELISA is always positive, but tends to remain positive even after cure and hence cannot indicate current disease. Colitis is often absent. On CXR there is elevation of the right hemidiaphragm. Treatment is with metronidazole.

Question 15 Cholestatic jaundice is not a recognized complication of:

A Isoniazid.
B Halothane.
C Chlorpromazine.
D Phenylbutazone.
E Norethandrolone.

Question 16 The following is not true of pernicious anaemia:

A Is associated with suppressed serum gastrin levels.
B 50% of patients have thyroid antibodies.
C Parietal cell antibodies are present in virtually all patients.
D Thrombocytopenia is a feature.
E Iron utilization is impaired.

Question 17 The following is not true of hepatitis C virus:

A Is a double stranded RNA virus.
B Acute infection is often subclinical.
C There is a significant risk of hepatocellular carcinoma.
D Blood transfusion has been an important source of transmission.
E PCR provides a direct measure of viral replication.

Answer 15

D Phenylbutazone.

Isoniazid and halothane cause an acute hepatitis.

Chlorpromazine and norethandrolone can induce an acute cholestasis. Liver biopsy shows intrahepatic cholestasis with eosinophilia.

Phenylbutazone causes granulomatous damage to the liver.

Drugs known to induce acute cholestasis are:
- Aspirin.
- Paracetamol.
- Isoniazid.
- Halothane.
- Antibiotics (penicillins, augmentin, and cephalosporins).
- Allopurinol.
- Cytotoxics (cyclophosphamide, vincristine).
- Hydralazine.
- Frusemide.
- Phenytoin.
- Methyldopa.
- MAO inhibitors.

Answer 16

A Is associated with suppressed serum gastrin levels.

In patients with pernicious anaemia, gastrin levels are usually very high and occur in response to achlorhydria. Parietal cell antibodies are present in nearly all patients, whereas intrinsic factor antibodies occur in approximately 50%. There is an association with other autoimmune disease, in particular thyroiditis, with thyroid antibodies present in 50% of patients. Adrenal antibodies may also be present. Iron utilization is impaired and purpura may arise as a result of thrombocytopenia.

Answer 17

A Is a double stranded RNA virus.

Hepatitis C is a single stranded RNA virus. Transmission is most frequently as a result of contaminated blood products, e.g. from transfusion or shared needles by drug addicts. Transmission by sexual intercourse and vertical transmission occur less frequently in comparison with hepatitis B infection. The incubation period is 6–12 weeks and infection is usually subclinical. Twenty-five percent of patients have jaundice, 50% develop chronic liver disease, 5% develop cirrhosis, and 15% of this group develop hepatocellular carcinoma. Antibody tests only become positive after 3–6 months and do not distinguish between infection and infectivity. Direct viral replication can be measured by PCR, and this can be used to monitor infection along with serum ALT. Treatment with interferon can suppress chronic infection.

Question 18 Accepted features of thiamine deficiency include:

A Dermatitis.
B Psoriasis.
C Glossitis.
D Wernicke's encephalopathy.
E Diarrhoea.

Question 19 The following statement about iron absorption is not true:

A Absorption is greatest in the duodenum and jejunum.
B In deficiency, absorption of iron dose is increased >threefold.
C Loss of iron from the body is 10 mg/day in the absence of menstruation.
D Intoxication by oral iron causes GI bleeding, liver failure, acidosis, and delayed liver failure.
E Serum levels show a diurnal variation.

Question 20 In the normal alimentary tract:

A Gastrin is secreted by gastric mucosal cells into the lumen of the stomach.
B Oxyntic cell activity is influenced by gastrin.
C Glucose is absorbed by simple diffusion.
D Gut motility is increased by vagal stimulation.
E B12 is absorbed in the duodenum after interaction with intrinsic factor.

Answer 18

D Wernicke's encephalopathy.

Thiamine deficiency is seen in areas of Asia where polished rice is consumed, with no fortification with thiamine. Polyneuropathy and Wernicke's encephalopathy are accepted features of thiamine deficiency.

Tutorial

In the western world, the condition is seen most frequently in malnourished chronic alcoholics. The resultant condition is known as beriberi. In dry beriberi there is axonal degeneration and demyelination, resulting in a sensorimotor polyneuropathy as well as muscle weakness and tenderness. Wernicke's encephalopathy is also seen in this group, which consists of a triad of ataxia, ophthalmoplegia, and amnesia syndrome. Wet beriberi is associated with oedema, ascites, pleural effusions, tachycardia, wide pulse pressure, and high output cardiac failure.

Dermatitis is a feature of riboflavin deficiency and also of niacin deficiency (pellagra). Glossitis is common in vitamin deficiencies but is not a feature of thiamine, but rather riboflavin deficiency, where it may occur in association with angular stomatitis. Diarrhoea is a feature of pellagra.

Answer 19

C Loss of iron from the body is 10 mg/day in the absence of menstruation.

Iron is absorbed in the duodenum and jejunum. It is transferred in the plasma bound to beta-globulin transferrin, which is synthesized in the liver. In the absence of menstruation, 0.5–1 mg is lost in faeces, urine, and sweat; an extra 0.7 mg is lost a day during menstruation. Serum levels show a diurnal variation, highest in the morning.

Answer 20

B Oxyntic cell activity is influenced by gastrin.

Gastrin is a hormone, which is secreted into the blood. Its release is particularly stimulated by protein ingestion and gastric distension. The main physiological action is the stimulation of gastric acid secretion.

B12 is absorbed in the ileum, glucose is absorbed actively.

7 Haematology

Question 1 The following are true of anaemia of chronic disease with the exception of:

A May complicate malignancy.
B The TIBC is reduced.
C The serum ferritin may be increased.
D In renal failure may respond to erythropoetin.
E May be complicated by a post-cricoid web.

Question 2 The following is true for sideroblastic anaemia:

A Inherited form is autosomal recessive.
B Is associated with iron deficiency.
C Ringed sideroblasts in the blood film are highly indicative of diagnosis.
D Is characteristically associated with a dimorphic blood film.
E May complicate treatment with rifampicin.

Question 3 Howell–Jolly bodies occur in:

A Uraemia.
B Sickle cell anaemia.
C Abetalipoproteinaemia.
D Pernicious anaemia.
E Lead poisoning.

Question 4 Vitamin B12:

A Is usually destroyed by cooking.
B Is a co-enzyme for thymidylate synthase.
C In the serum is mainly bound to albumin.
D Is activated by nitric oxide.
E Is reduced in chronic myeloid leukaemia.

Question 5 Macrocytic anaemia may complicate the following with the exception of:

A *Ancyclostoma duodenale* infestation.
B Treatment with zidovudine.
C Treatment with phenytoin.
D Hypothyroidism.
E Thymic tumour.

Answer 1

E May be complicated by a post-cricoid web.

Anaemia of chronic disease may complicate infection, malignancy, connective tissue diseases (SLE, RA), Crohn's, and chronic renal failure. Typically there is:

- A mild normocytic anaemia (Hb >8).
- Reduced TIBC (raised in iron deficiency).
- Reduced serum iron.
- Normal or raised serum ferritin which distinguishes it from iron deficiency anaemia.
- Iron stores are normal and hence the anaemia does not respond to iron therapy.

In chronic renal failure erythropoetin is frequently used to correct anaemia. Side-effects include 'flu'-like illness, hypertension, and increased platelet count.

Answer 2

D Is characteristically associated with a dimorphic blood film.

Sideroblastic anaemia may be congenital or acquired. Congenital cases are rare and X-linked. Most cases are idiopathic. The condition is characterized with iron overload and dyserythropoiesis.

Sideroblasts are erythroblasts with iron deposited in a ring around the nucleus which can be demonstrated using a prussian blue stain. They are found in the bone marrow. The blood film shows a dimorphic picture with the presence of both normal and microcytic cells.

Acquired causes include:

- Alcohol.
- Drugs (isoniazid).
- Malabsorption.
- Malignancy.
- Myeloproliferative disorders.
- Leukaemia.
- Lead poisoning.
- Connective tissue diseases.

Complications include iron deposition in the liver, myocardium, and endocrine glands. Treatment is supportive. The patient should be advised to stop adverse medication/alcohol. Pyridoxine and folic acid may improve iron utilization.

Answer 3

B Sickle cell anaemia.

Howell–Jolly bodies are nucleur remnants seen in RBCs. They are seen in:

- Iron deficiency anaemia.
- Post-splenectomy (or splenic atrophy as in coeliac disease, sickle cell anaemia).
- Megaloblastic anaemia.
- Leukaemia.

Burr cells (irregularly shaped RBCs) are seen in uraemia. Acanthocytes (spiculated RBCs) occur in abetalipoproteinaemia.

Lead poisoning is associated with:

- Hypochromic or haemolytic anaemia.
- Basophilic stippling of RBCs.
- Ring sideroblasts in the bone marrow.

Answer 4

B Is a co-enzyme for thymidylate synthase.

The average diet contains 15–30 µg a day of vitamin B12, of which 1–5 µg are absorbed. Stores are sufficient to last 3–5 years before deficiency becomes apparent.

The structure of B12 is based on a planar group with a central cobalt atom referred to as a corrin ring. B12 is a co-enzyme for thymidylate synthase which is necessary for DNA synthesis (for conversion of methyltetrahydrofolate to N5,N10-methylene tetrahydrofolate). In the serum, 90% of B12 is bound to transcobalamin I and 10% to transcobalamin III. These cobalamins are derived from granulocytes and as a result B12 is increased in myeloproliferative disorders.

Vitamin B12 is not destroyed by cooking but it is inactivated by nitric oxide.

Answer 5

E Thymic tumour.

This question frequently features as 'causes of megaloblastic anaemia' so we aim to cover all aspects in this answer. Megaloblastic anaemia is caused by folate and B12 deficiency. Ancyclostoma (hookworm) infection is associated with a hypochromic, microcytic anaemia.

Tutorial

Causes of folate deficiency:
- Poor dietary intake.
- Alcoholism.
- Old age.
- Starvation.
- Malabsorption:
  - Coeliac disease.
  - Crohn's disease.
  - Partial gastrectomy.
  - Gastrointestinal malignancy.
- Excess utilization:
  - Pregnancy, lactation.
  - Prematurity.
- Excess red cell production, e.g. haemolysis.
- Haemodialysis/CAPD.
- Drugs:
  - Phenytoin.
  - Primidone.
  - Methotrexate.

Causes of vitamin B12 deficiency:
- Dietary (vegans).
- Gastrointestinal:
  - Pernicious anaemia.
  - Gastrectomy.
  - Coeliac disease.
  - Tropical sprue.
  - Bacterial overgrowth.
  - Ileal resection.
  - Chronic pancreatitis.
  - Zollinger–Ellison syndrome.
  - Fish tapeworm.

Causes of macrocytosis without megaloblastic anaemia:
- Hypothyroidism.
- Reticulocytosis (haemolysis).
- Liver disease.
- Aplastic anaemia.
- Pregnancy.
- Zidovudine.
- Azathioprine.

Question 6 The following is not true with reference to hereditary spherocytosis:

A Inheritance is autosomal dominant.
B May be complicated by megaloblastic crises.
C Leg ulceration is a feature.
D Osmotic fragility is reduced.
E Splenectomy is the treatment of choice.

Question 7 Haemolytic anaemia:

A Is not caused by pyruvate kinase deficiency.
B Does not occur in beta-thalassaemia.
C Is associated with reduced serum haptoglobin.
D Is not a recognized complication of treatment with mefanamic acid.
E The Donnath–Landsteiner antibody is protective against haemolysis.

Answer 6

D Osmotic fragility is reduced.

Hereditary spherocytosis is inherited as an autosomal dominant trait with incomplete penetrance. The resultant RBC has several abnormalities:
- Defect in structural protein septrin.
- Reduced surface area to volume ratio.
- Increased permeability to sodium ions.

Clinical features:
- Neonatal jaundice – in some cases only.
- Anaemia.
- Splenomegaly.
- Leg ulcers (more common in adults).
- Bone hypertrophy typically affecting the skull and maxillary sinuses.
- Haemolysis.
- Pigment gall stones.

Infection may precipitate an aplastic crisis. The marrow is hyperactive resulting in folate deficiency and hence increasing the possibility of megaloblastic crisis.

Investigations show:
- Anaemia.
- Blood film: spherocytes, macrocytes, and reticulocytes.
- Increased serum bilirubin and urine urobilinogen (haemolysis).
- Osmotic fragility.
- Negative direct Coombs' test.

Treatment:
- Splenectomy in all but the mildest cases.
- Spherocytes persist but Hb returns to normal and red cells are no longer prematurely lysed.

Other causes of spherocytes on blood film:
- Infection.
- Burns.
- Haemolysis.

Answer 7

C Is associated with reduced serum haptoglobin.

Haemolysis is said to occur when the mean RBC survival is <120 days. If the bone marrow is unable to compensate, there will be a resultant anaemia.

Evidence for haemolysis:
- Increased serum bilirubin and urinary urobilinogen.
- Reduced plasma haptoglobin.
- Abnormal red cell fragments in the blood film.
- Reticulocytosis (due to increased red cell production).

Tutorial

Causes of haemolytic anaemia
Membrane abnormalities:
- Hereditary spherocytosis (above).
- Hereditary elliptocytosis: AD, similar to hereditary spherocytosis but the cells are elliptical. Haemolysis is usually mild and only a few patients have anaemia.

  Splenectomy is indicated where anaemia occurs.

Haemoglobinopathies:
- Sickle cell anaemia.
- Thalassaemia.

Enzyme disorders:
- Pyruvate kinase deficiency: autosomal recessive, homozygotes present with neonatal jaundice. The enzyme catalyses the conversion of 1,3 DPG to 3-PG (glycolytic pathway). The disorder becomes more chronic with advancing age, with chronic haemolysis, jaundice, and splenomegaly. Pyruvate kinase activity is shown to be significantly reduced.

  Chronic anaemia and the rise in intra-cellular 2,3 DPG shift the oxygen dissociation curve. Reticulocytosis and altered cell shape are seen on blood films. A high rate of autohaemolysis occurs which is not altered by the addition of glucose to RBCs, which distinguishes it from hereditary spherocytosis. Splenectomy is considered where anaemia is symptomatic.
- Glucose-6-phosphate dehydrogenase deficiency: the commonest RBC enzyme defect. Inheritance is sex linked (the gene is carried on the X chromosome), and is increased in males. Female carriers show markedly reduced enzyme levels in their RBCs. It is common in Africa, the Mediterranean, the Middle East, and south east Asia.

  The enzyme catalyses the conversion of glucose to glucose-6-phosphate. The majority of cases are asymptomatic but are susceptible to oxidative crises which may occur in response to drugs or infection. Presentation occurs as neonatal jaundice or oxidative crisis.

Agents precipitating oxidative crisis:

- Fava beans (does not occur in varient G6PD deficiency).
- Acute illness (DKA).
- Infection.
- Drugs:
  – Antimalarials: quinine, primaquine, pyrimethamine, chloroquine.
  – Analgesics: aspirin, phenacetin.
  – Antibacterials: sulphonamides, dapsone, nitrofurantoin, chloramphenicol.
  – Other: vitamin K, probenacid, quinidine.

The blood count in between attacks is normal. During attacks there is evidence of haemolysis, reticulocytosis, and Heinz bodies (denatured haemoglobin; stained with methyl violet). Treatment is removal of the offending drug and occasionally blood transfusion. There is no role for splenectomy in the treatment.

Drug-induced immune haemolysis:

- Due to antigenic effects on RBC membranes, e.g. penicillin.
- Due to development of RBC autoantibodies, e.g. methyldopa, mefanamic acid, L-dopa.

Autoimmune haemolytic anaemia:

- Warm: may present with acute or chronic anaemia. Treatment is with steroids or splenectomy.
- Cold: may occur following mycoplasma infection. Treatment is to advise the patient to keep warm. Chlorambucil has been used with satisfactory results.

The Donnath–Landsteiner antibody causes paroxysmal cold haemoglobinuria which is a well recognized cause of haemolytic anaemia. It occurs following infection with mumps, chickenpox, syphilis, and measles. Haemolysis is due to complement-mediated lysis.

Other causes of haemolytic anaemia include:

- Trauma from prosthetic heart valves especially aortic.
- Microangiopathic haemolytic anaemia caused by septicaemia.
- DIC.
- Haemolytic uraemic syndrome.
- Thrombotic thrombocytopenia purpura.
- Polyarteritis nodosa.
- Malignant hypertension.
- Giant haemangioma.
- Paroxysmal nocturnal haemoglobinuria (covered later).

Question 8 An adult with sickle cell anaemia may have the following complication:

A Splenomegaly.
B Leg ulcers.
C Septic necrosis of the bone.
D Dysphagia.
E Sterility.

Question 9 The following is not true for beta-thalassaemia major:

A HbF is characteristically elevated.
B Splenomegaly is a feature.
C Iron loading is exacerbated by administration of dexferroxamine.
D Cardiac siderosis is an important cause of death.
E Bone X-rays show a classical 'hair on end' appearance.

Question 10 The following are necessary for the diagnosis of homozygous beta-thalassaemia with the exception of:

A Hypochromia.
B Absent adult HbA_2.
C Increased HbF.
D Normal or high serum iron.
E Megaloblasts in the marrow.

Answer 8

B Leg ulcers.

Adults with sickle cell anaemia suffer from numerous complications including:

- Dactylitis due to microinfarction, more common in childhood.
- Aseptic necrosis affecting the femoral heads in particular; secondary to bone infarction.
- Osteomyelitis frequently due to salmonella.
- Chronic leg ulcers usually on the medial surface of the lower tibia.
- Pulmonary fibrosis with pulmonary hypertension.
- Iron overload from recurrent blood transfusion.
- Papillary necrosis of the kidney causing haematuria.
- Painful priapism.

The spleen is usually not palpable due to recurrent infarction. Dysphagia and sterility are not features. Pregnancy does increase the possibility of crisis. Children with sickle cell may have splenomegaly and even hepatosplenomegaly due to sequestration. Hand and foot syndrome is common in children and manifests with painful swelling of the digits of the hands and feet.

Answer 9

C Iron loading is exacerbated by administration of dexferroxamine.

In beta-thalassaemia major iron overload due to recurrent transfusion results in deposition of iron in the myocardium, endocrine glands, and liver. Cardiac siderosis is an important cause of death. Desferroxamine infusions assist in preventing iron overload. Features of this condition include:

- Failure to thrive.
- Growth retardation.
- Severe anaemia.
- Skeletal deformity with frontal bossing.
- Splenomegaly.
- Bleeding.
- Intermittent fever.
- X-rays show characteristic ‘hair on end’ appearance.

Answer 10

E Megaloblasts in the marrow.

In beta-thalassaemia haemoglobin electrophoresis shows:

- Very high HbF.
- Absent adult HbA.
- Variable HbA_2.

There is a moderate to severe anaemia with decreasing MCV and MCH. The reticulocyte count is increased. The blood film shows a hypochromic, microcytic picture and Howell–Jolly bodies may be present due to hyposplenism. TIBC (total iron binding capacity) is saturated, with high ferritin levels due to multiple transfusions.

Question 11 The following is true for haemophilia A:

A Is inherited as an X-linked dominant trait.
B The gene is located on the Y chromosome.
C The bleeding time is increased.
D Factor IX is depleted.
E The PTTK is increased.

Question 12 The following statement regarding haemophilia A in a 6-year-old child is correct:

A Melaena is a frequent complication.
B Haematuria is more likely to be due to renal disease than haemophilia.
C All his brothers will be haemophiliacs.
D Knee haemarthroses should always be aspirated.
E A factor VIII concentrate should be given to arrest haemorrhage.

Question 13 If a child suffers from factor IX deficiency, the disorder of blood clotting is also seen in:

A His father.
B His sisters.
C His father's brothers.
D His mother's brothers.
E His sisters.

Question 14 A male aged 32 years has haemarthroses with a prolonged PTTK, normal PT, and a normal bleeding time. He is likely to have:

A Henoch–Schönlein syndrome.
B Factor X deficiency.
C Factor VII deficiency.
D Factor VIII deficiency.
E von Willebrand's disease.

Question 15 Acute lymphoblastic leukaemia:

A Is associated with maternal exposure to sawdust.
B Is more common in Down's syndrome.
C Bleeding is uncommon.
D The bone marrow is hypocellular.
E Is more common in adult males.

Answer 11

E The PTTK is increased.

Haemophilia A is inherited as an X-linked recessive (the gene is located on the long arm of chromosome X). The bleeding time is normal, factor VIII:C is depleted, the PTTK is increased.

Factor IX is depleted in haemophilia B (Christmas disease). The inheritance and clinical manifestations are identical to haemophilia A. Female carriers have a tendency to increased bleeding.

Answer 12

E A factor VIII concentrate should be given to arrest haemorrhage.

Haemophilia A is characterized by depletion of factor VIII:C which has coagulant activity. The other component (VIII:Ag which is associated with platelet function), is normal. Inheritance is X-linked recessive, hence some of his brothers may be affected and some of his sisters may be carriers.

The most severely affected individuals have factor VIII levels $<2\%$. Haemorrhage into joints is often spontaneous and may be complicated by severe arthropathy. These should not be aspirated but treated with factor VIII infusion to stop bleeding, increasing levels to $>50\%$ of normal. Trauma may result in bleeding into muscles, neck, or kidneys resulting in haematomas and nerve compressions, leading to palsies. Life threatening haemorrhage causing airways obstruction requires factor VIII infusions to raise the level to $>100\%$ of normal.

Answer 13

D His mother's brothers.

Females are the carriers and only males are affected.

Answer 14

D Factor VIII deficiency.

The male is likely to have factor IX or VIII deficiency. In haemophilia A (factor VIII:C deficiency) and haemophilia B (factor IX deficiency):

- Bleeding time is normal.
- PTTK is increased.
- PT is normal.

In von Willebrand's disease, there is a reduced level of all factor VIII components, resulting in:

- Bleeding time is increased.
- PTTK is increased.
- PT is normal.

Answer 15

B Is more common in Down's syndrome.

ALL is the commonest childhood leukaemia which is more common in males. ALL is more common in children than in adults. The exact cause of ALL is not known, although there is an association with:
- Preconception exposure to paternal radiation, sawdust.
- Benzene.
- Drugs, e.g. phenylbutazone.
- HTLV-1 virus.

The condition is more common in patients with Down's syndrome.

Clinical features are due to marrow failure, and include:
- Anaemia.
- Acute oral cavity infections, ulceration, and pneumonia.
- Tender lymphadenopathy.
- Splenomegaly and thymic enlargement.
- Bleeding and bruising.
- Bone pain and arthritis.
- Gum hypertrophy due to tissue infiltration.
- Increased ICP and cranial nerve palsies.

Investigations show:
- Hypercellular bone marrow with characteristic blast cells.
- Normochromic, normocytic anaemia.
- Thrombocytopenia.

Poor prognostic features include:
- Age <2 or >10 years.
- High initial leucocyte count.
- CNS involvement.
- Thymic enlargement.
- Massive hepatosplenomegaly and lymphadenopathy.
- Presence of T- and B-cell markers on the blast cells.

Question 16 The following is not true for acute myeloid leukaemia:

A Characteristically results in death within 2 months if untreated.
B May complicate chemotherapy for other haematological malignancies.
C Proptosis is a recognized feature.
D Is associated with the Philadelphia chromosome.
E Splenomegaly is a feature.

Question 17 The following is not true for hairy cell leukaemia:

A B-cell leukaemias are more common than T-cell.
B Blood film usually consists of a leucoerythroblastic picture.
C Massive splenomegaly is a recognized feature.
D May respond to splenectomy.
E Does respond to interferon.

Question 18 The following is true for chronic lymphatic leukaemia:

A Thrombocytopenia is associated with a good prognosis.
B Hepatosplenomegaly is an early feature.
C Coombs'-positive haemolysis is a recognized feature.
D Immunoglobulins are markedly raised.
E Cellular immunity is not preserved.

Answer 16

D Is associated with the Philadelphia chromosome.

AML is one of the most rapidly progressing haematological malignancies, resulting in death if not treated within 2 months. It affects 1/10 000 and increases with age. It is a recognized complication of long-term chemotherapy, e.g. for lymphoma.

Clinical features are due to:

- Marrow failure.
- Anaemia.
- Infection, often Gram-negative.
- Bleeding.
- Leukaemic infiltration.
- Bone pain, tender sternum.
- CNS infiltration, cranial nerve palsies, cord compression.
- Gum hypertrophy, proptosis due to orbital infiltration.
- Testicular tenderness.
- Lymphadenopathy, hepatosplenomegaly.
- Proptosis may be caused by infiltration of the ocular muscles.

Blast cells contain granules which amalgamate to form au$_r$ rods which differentiate the cells from ALL. White cell thrombi (leucostasis) are well recognized and lead to pulmonary and cerebral infarcts.

Answer 17

B Blood film usually consists of a leucoerythroblastic picture.

Hairy cell leukemia is a rare haematological malignancy, characterized by blast cells which have spiculated cytoplasmic surfaces giving a 'hairy' appearance. Most malignancies are of the B-cell type. The blood film usually demonstrates a pancytopenia and there is associated massive splenomegaly.

Splenectomy may cause remission for a period of months to years but this condition is resistant to usual specific therapy for leukaemia. It has been shown to respond to interferon and deoxycoformycin.

Answer 18

C Coombs'-positive haemolysis is a recognized feature.

Chronic lymphatic leukaemia is a disease of middle/old age consisting of monoclonal proliferation of well-differentiated lymphocytes. More than 99% are B-cell malignancies. It is twice as common in men, constituting 25% of all leukaemias.

Tutorial

Symptoms of chronic lymphatic leukaemia:

- 25% have none.
- Lethargy.
- Fever and sweating.
- Anorexia and weight loss.
- Bleeding.

Signs:

- Nontender lymphadenopathy in the neck, axilla, and groin.
- Late hepatosplenomegaly.
- Skin infiltration with intense itching (*l'homme rouge*).

Investigations show:

- Normochromic, normocytic anaemia.
- Marked lymphocytosis.
- Thrombocytopenia.
- Evidence for haemolysis.

Anaemia may acutely deteriorate due to Coombs'-positive haemolysis.

Staging uses the Rai staging system (staging correlates with survival):

O = Absolute lymphocytosis $>15 \times 10^9$/l.
I = Stage O + enlarged lymph nodes.
II = Stage I + enlarged liver or spleen.
III = Stage II + anaemia Hb <11 g/dl.
IV = Stage III + thrombocytopenia platelets $<100 \times 10^9$/l.

Complications:

- Autoimmune haemolysis.
- Hypogammaglobulinaemia with predominant reduction in IgM.
- Immune paresis.
- Bacterial infection.
- 2% acute lymphoblastic transformation.
- 10% develop histiocytic lymphoma.
- 20% of cases are complicated by herpes zoster infection.

Cellular immunity is usually preserved. Patients with early disease do not usually require treatment. When symptoms occur, treatment with chlorambucil is effective. Other useful drugs are cyclophosphamide and prednisolone. Avoid radiotherapy in early disease as it may precipitate marrow failure, unless there is a specific indication, e.g. mediastinal obstruction. Vaccination with vaccinia is contraindicated due to the risks of vaccinia.

Other causes of positive direct Coombs' test include:

- Gangrenosum.
- SLE.
- α-methyldopa therapy.
- Lymphoma.
- Malignancy.

Question 19 The following is true for chronic myeloid leukaemia:

A The presence of the Philadelphia chromosome is associated with a worse prognosis.
B Priapism is a recognized feature.
C Leucocyte alkaline phosphatase levels are raised.
D Serum folate levels are increased.
E Lymphadenopathy is common.

Question 20 Hodgkin's lymphoma:

A Is associated with tender lymphadenopathy.
B Persistent low grade pyrexia is typical.
C Alcohol consumption is associated with flushing.
D Thrombocytopenia is a common feature.
E Is confirmed histologically by the presence of Reed–Sternberg cells.

Question 21 The following may indicate underlying malignant lymphoma with the exception of:

A Acquired ichthyosis.
B Chronic discoid lupus erythmatosis.
C Herpes zoster.
D Alcohol induced pain at the site of lymphadenopathy.
E Generalized pruritis.

Answer 19

B Priapism is a recognized feature.

In patients with CML, the Philadelphia chromosome is present in >95% of granulocyte, RBC, and platelet precursors. The Philadelphia chromosome is chromosome 22 which has lost 50% of its long arm. In nearly all cases this is translocated to the long arm of chromosome 9. Its presence is characterized by relatively slow progression of disease, whereas its absence is associated with a particularly bad prognosis.

Tutorial

Symptoms of CML:
- Insidious onset of fatigue, due to anaemia.
- LUQ discomfort from massive splenomegaly.
- Sweating and fever due to hypermetabolism.
- Bleeding and bruising.

Signs:
- Pallor.
- Massive splenomegaly.
- Lymphadenopathy is uncommon.
- Priapism.
- Gout.

Investigations show:
- Hb may be normal or normochromic, normocytic anaemia.
- WCC >50 × 10^9/l (film: excess neutrophils with myelocytes and blast cells).
- Platelets may be increased.
- Leucocyte ALP is very low.
- B12 is increased.

Treatment is with busulphan and hydroxyurea.

Answer 20

E Is confirmed histologically by the presence of Reed–Sternberg cells.

Hodgkin's disease commonly presents with enlarged nontender cervical lymphadenopathy. Fever and sweating are common, but the classical Pel–Ebstein fever consists of a few days of high pyrexia alternating with a few days of apyrexia. Alcohol consumption is associated with pain in the lymph nodes *not* flushing, which occurs in carcinoid.

FBC may be normal in early disease, but later there is:
- Normochromic, normocytic anaemia.
- Increased ESR.
- Leucoerythroblastic anaemia (marrow infiltration).
- Increased WCC and eosinophilia.

There may be associated hypercalcaemia, hyperuricaemia, and deranged LFTs. CXR may show mediastinal lymphadenopathy.

Reed–Sternberg cells are diagnostic and consist of mirror image nuclei.

Histological classification:
- Nodular sclerosing: good prognosis.
- Mixed cellularity: good prognosis.
- Lymphocyte predominant: good prognosis.
- Lymphocyte depleted: poor prognosis.

Answer 21

B Chronic discoid lupus erythmatosis.

Ichthyosis is often a congenital condition usually present at birth, in which the skin is dry, rough, and scaly because of a defect in keratinization. It may however be a cutaneous manifestation of lymphoma.

Discoid lupus is a benign variant of systemic lupus erythematosis where skin involvement is the only feature. The lesions are well demarcated erythematous plaques which in time cause scarring and pigmentation of the area affected. This is not, however, the rule and in some instances systemic abnormalities may occur with time. Herpes zoster frequently complicates conditions that are associated with impaired immunity.

Pruritis is a generalized symptom which may complicate many infective and metabolic conditions. Pruritis associated with fever, night sweats, and alcohol-induced pain at the site of lymphadenopathy should alert one to the possible diagnosis of lymphoma.

Question 22 The following are features of polcythaemia rubra vera with the exception of:

A Gastrointestinal haemorrhage.
B Increased leucocyte alkaline phosphatase.
C Reduced arterial oxygen saturation.
D Hyperuricaemia.
E Thrombocythaemia.

Question 23 Myeloma may be complicated by the following with the exception of:

A Central retinal vein occlusion.
B Bone tenderness.
C Amyloidosis.
D Premature death if Hb <7.5 g/dl.
E Lucent bone lesions on X-ray.

Question 24 Amyloid disease is a recognized complication of the following with the exception of:

A Traumatic paraplegia.
B Leprosy.
C Rheumatoid arthritis.
D Familial Mediterranean fever.
E Thalassaemia.

Answer 22

C Reduced arterial oxygen saturation.

Polycythaemia rubra vera is more common in patients >60 years of age.

Symptoms include:
- Fatigue.
- Vertigo and tinnitus.
- Angina and claudication.
- Haemorrhagic tendencies.
- Itching, particularly after a hot bath or in a warm enviroment.
- Gout due to increased cell turnover.

Patients are plethoric with injected conjunctiva. Hepatosplenomegaly is common.

Investigations show:
- PCV >0.55.
- Hb >18 g/dl.
- Increased platelet and WCC.
- Increased serum uric acid.
- Increased leucocyte ALP.
- Increased serum B12.

Treatment is with venesection to keep PCV <50%. Intravenous ^{32}P or busulphan may be effective. Polycythaemia frequently progresses to myelosclerosis or AML.

Secondary polycythaemia may be caused by:
- Smoking.
- COPD.
- Hypernephroma.
- Hepatoma.
- Fibroids.
- Altitude.

Stress polycythaemia (Gaisbocks syndrome): a condition affecting overweight hypertensive men who smoke. The red cell volume is normal but the plasma volume is reduced, resulting in a relative polycythaemia. Venesection is advised to normalize PCV and patients should be strongly advised not to smoke.

Answer 23

E Lucent bone lesions on X-ray.

Myeloma is a hyperviscosity state which may predispose to vascular occlusion. Bony involvement may result in tenderness and pathological fracture.

Answer 24

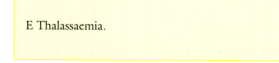

E Thalassaemia.

Amyloid is a homogenous hyaline-like substance which stains pink with H&E, red with congo red and is apple green under polarized light. It is classified according to the nature of the protein involved.

AL amyloid: consists of light chains and may be primary. It may complicate lymphoproliferative disease, e.g.:
- Myeloma.
- Waldenstrom's macroglobulinaemia.
- Non-Hodgkin's lymphoma.

Macroglossia is characteristic. Patients may present with cardiac failure or nephrotic syndrome (depending on the organs involved).

Hepatomegaly, purpura, and bleeding are common, but splenomegaly is rare.

AA amyloid (reactive systemic amyloidosis): involves the spleen, kidney, liver, and adrenals. It is associated with chronic infection and inflammation e.g.:
- Leprosy/TB.
- Rheumatoid arthritis.
- Malignancy (Hodgkin's disease).
- Familial Mediterranean fever.

It is also seen in chronic paraplegia.

8 Infectious Diseases

Question 1 The following is true of rabies infection:

A It is caused by a DNA virus.
B The incubation period is 14 days.
C Behavioural disturbances do not occur.
D CSF shows a reduced protein.
E Hydrophobia is characteristic of furious rabies.

Question 2 Side-effects of zidovudine do not include:

A Agranulocytosis.
B Paraesthesia.
C Nail pigmentation.
D Drowsiness.
E Myopathy.

Question 3 The following infection is not associated with eosinophilia:

A *Ascaris lumbricoides*.
B Filaria.
C Schistosomiasis.
D Amoebiasis.
E Toxocara.

Question 4 The following statement is true of schistosomiasis:

A *S. mansoni* most commonly affects the bladder.
B Most infections are acquired at midday.
C The severity of disease is related to the extent of replication of adult schistosomes in the host.
D Portal hypertension with variceal bleeding is not a recognized complication.
E There is a significant association with carcinoma of the bladder.

Answer 1

E Hydrophobia is characteristic of furious rabies.

Rabies is caused by a single stranded bullet shaped RNA virus of the Rhabdoviridae group. The incubation period varies from 7 days to several years but is <60 days in 70% of patients. Prodromal symptoms herald the symptoms of rabies by 2–7 days, and consist of fever, malaise, sore throat, cough, myalgia, headache, and diarrhoea. Behavioural disturbances frequently occur, and consist of agitation, aggression, and intolerance to tactile auditory and visual stimuli.

Tutorial

CSF:
- Normal opening pressure.
- Mixed pleocytosis.
- Protein is slightly raised in 25% of patients in week 1, but rises to 100 mg/dl.

Furious rabies: triad of hyperexcitability, painful muscle spasms, and hydrophobia.

Dumb rabies: features are of ascending paralysis preceded by paraesthesia localized to the site of the bite.

Answer 2

D Drowsiness.

Zidovudine causes myelosuppression, and hence anaemia, neutropenia, leucopenia, and pancytopenia, which are more common on higher doses.

Paraesthesia, myopathy, nail and mucosal pigmentation are well documented. Zidovudine may cause insomnia. It also produces fatty change in the liver with associated hepatomegaly and lactic acidosis.

Tutorial

Mechanism of action
In vitro, zidovudine has been shown to inhibit the replication of HIV-1, HIV-2, and HTLV-1. It is used in combination with interferon alpha to treat HTLV-1 infection. Zidovudine has also been shown to reduce vertical transmission of HIV infection by up to 50% when used in the last trimester of pregnancy.

Resistance to AZT and other retroviral drugs is mediated by mutations on the *pol* gene encoding for the reverse transcriptase enzyme.

Answer 3

D Amoebiasis.

Eosinophilia is usually suggestive of an underlying parasitic infection and is most frequently seen in helminthic infections. It usually occurs during the migratory phase of such infections, which explains why patients with established infections often have a normal eosinophil count.

Other infective causes of eosinophilia include:
- Cysticercus.
- Echinococcus.
- Filaria.
- Strongyloides.
- Trichinella.
- *Trichus trichuria*.

Answer 4

B Most infections are acquired at midday.

Schistosomes are trematodes or flatworms. The vector is the fresh water snail. Infected snails release up to 1000 cercariae a day, which penetrate the skin of the host from the water. Release of cercariae is stimulated by daylight and warmth, and water densities are highest at midday. Tissue damage results from egg deposition. There is no replication in the host.

Tutorial

S. mansoni and *S. japonicum* cause intestinal schistosomiasis, which is associated with:

- Malabsorption (osteomalacia).
- Persistent bloody diarrhoea.
- Granulomatous liver disease with cirrhosis.
- Portal hypertension, hepatosplenomegaly, and varices.

Liver function is usually well preserved.

S. haematobium preferentially affects the vesical venous plexus with resultant urogenital system involvement causing:

- Haematuria, dysuria, and suprapubic pain.
- Obstructive uropathy with calculus formation and secondary infection.
- Bladder calcification, ulceration, papilloma, and carcinoma.
- Lesions on the cervix.

The eggs are often found on rectal biopsy.

In acute infection there is a fever, diarrhoea, vomiting, weight loss, and possible CNS and pulmonary involvement, resulting in a sacral radiculitis, which may progress to transverse myelitis. The treatment of choice is praziquantel. Side-effects include abdominal pain and urticarial rash, most commonly occurring around lips and eyes.

Katayama fever is an acute illness, characterized by fever, myalgia, and pulmonary infiltrates with eosinophilia, which occurs as a host response to egg production by the adult worms.

Question 5 Regarding infection with *Treponema pallidum*:

A The primary lesion is associated with tender regional lymphadenopathy.
B Sore throat is common in secondary syphilis.
C Gummatous lesions do not respond well to penicillin.
D Lymphogranuloma venerum is characteristic of tertiary syphilis.
E A baby born to an infected and adequately treated mother should be treated for infection if serological tests remain positive in the cord blood.

Question 6 The following condition is not associated with false positive tests for syphilis:

A Sjögren’s syndrome.
B Autoimmune haemolytic anaemia.
C SLE.
D Molluscum contagiosum.
E Myasthenia gravis.

Question 7 Infectious mononucleosis is not associated with:

A Atypical lymphocytes, which are not specific to this condition.
B Palatal petechiae.
C Autoimmune haemolytic anaemia.
D Mononeuritis multiplex.
E Positive *Treponema pallidum* immobilization test.

Answer 5

B Sore throat is common in secondary syphilis.

Primary disease occurs 2–4 weeks after exposure to *Treponema pallidum* and is associated with the development of a papule on the penis, vulva, cervix, or anus following close sexual contact. This ulcerates and becomes hard and painless and is associated with nontender regional lymphadenopathy.

Secondary syphilis occurs 2–3 months after the chancre has healed. It is associated with sore throat, malaise, fever, generalized lymphadenopathy, a nonitchy maculopapular rash, snail track ulcers affecting the mucous membranes, and condylomata lata occurring in the groin and perianal regions. The rashes of secondary syphilis spare the face but do affect the palms and soles. Patients may occasionally develop patchy alopecia and iritis.

Gummatous lesions occur in tertiary syphilis, affecting the skin, bones (especially skull, tibia, fibula), and visceral organs, especially liver (hepar lobatum). Syphilitic meningitis and gummatous lesions respond well to penicillin. Nerve deafness and interstitial keratitis respond less favourably.

Tutorial

Cardiovascular complications of syphilis include:
- Aortitis.
- Cardiac ischaemia, secondary to coronary ostial stenosis.
- Aortic incompetence.
- Aortic aneurysm.
- Heart block.

Neurological complications include:
- Tabes dorsalis (Argyll Robertson pupils, lightening pains, paraesthesia due to involvement of the posterior columns).
- GPI (cerebral cortex affected).
- Meningovascular syphilis (low grade meningitis).
- Neuropathy and perforating ulcers of the feet (other causes of these ulcers include diabetes and leprosy).

Active disease in the newborn is confirmed by demonstrating IgM antibodies in the cord blood, necessitating treatment. Treatment of tertiary syphilis is associated rarely with severe Jarisch–Herxheimer reaction, which occurs in 90% of patients with secondary syphilis to a much milder degree.

Lymphogranuloma venerum is due to *Chlamydia trachomatis* infection.

Answer 6

D Molluscum contagiosum.

Treponema pallidum haemagglutination assay (TPHA) is specific for treponemal infection. False positive reactions occur with other spirochaetal infections such as yaws, pinta, Lyme disease, and leptospirosis.

Tutorial

Venereal Disease Research Laboratory (VDRL) test is a nontreponemal test based on the detection of IgG and IgM antibodies to cardiolipin. Cardiolipin antibody tests such as Widal reaction (WR) and VDRL are positive in the serum in the great majority of untreated secondary, tertiary, and latent syphilis, but biological false positives can occur (above).

False positive results may be seen in:
- Recent immunization, e.g. smallpox vaccination.
- Pneumonitis (bacterial or viral pneumonia).
- Malaria.
- Infectious mononucleosis.
- Viral hepatitis.
- Mycoplasma.
- Cirrhosis.
- Malignancy.

More specific tests include TPI (*Treponema pallidum* immobilization) which remains positive for years after successful treatment, but is expensive and is now replaced by FTA (fluorescent treponema antibodies). FTA is positive in 90% of patients with primary disease and remains positive for life even after treatment. Activity on the VDRL correlates more closely with active infection.

Answer 7

E Positive *Treponema pallidum* immobilization test.

A common feature of infectious mononucleosis (glandular fever) is palatal petechiae. Autoimmune haemolytic anaemia occurs less commonly.

Tutorial

Common features of infectious mononucleosis include:
- Headache, fever, sore throat.
- Palatal petechiae.
- Tender cervical lymphadenopathy.
- Splenomegaly.
- Hepatitis.

Less common features are:

Haematological:
- Autoimmune haemolytic anaemia.
- Thrombocytopenia.
- Granulocytopenia.
- Eosinophilia.
- Mesenteric adenitis.

Cardiological:
- Pericarditis.
- Myocarditis and arrhythmias.

Pulmonary:
- Interstitial pneumonitis.
- Pleuretic chest pain.

Neurological:
- Encephalitis/meningoencephalitis.
- Cranial nerve palsy, especially Bell's palsy.
- Guillain–Barré syndrome.
- Mononeuritis multiplex.
- Transverse myelitis.
- Psychosis.

Atypical lymphocytes are also seen in infection with :
- CMV.
- Toxoplasmosis.
- Influenza.
- Rubella.
- HIV.

Vesicular rashes are not a feature of this condition. It occurs mainly in young adults. Heterophile antibodies occur in 30% of patients in week 1 and 90% of patients in week 2, and persist into convalescence.

Question 8 The following is true of infection with *Salmonella typhi*:

A Infection is spread from infected poultry.
B It is associated with a Pel Ebstein fever.
C Patients often have a resting tachycardia.
D Splenomegaly is not common.
E Co-trimoxazole is effective treatment.

Question 9 The following is not true for leptospirosis:

A Is caused by a spirochaete.
B Conjunctival suffusion is common.
C CSF protein content is increased.
D Jaundice is unusual.
E Jarisch–Herxheimer reaction may complicate treatment.

Answer 8

E Co-trimoxazole is effective treatment.

Salmonella typhi is a Gram-negative bacillus. Spread is by the faecal–oral route. The incubation period is 10–14 days. Humans are the only known reservoir for infection (remember Typhoid Mary)!

Tutorial

Symptoms occur in week 1 and consist of:
- Insidious headache.
- Nonproductive cough.
- Constipation.
- Abdominal pain.
- Confusion (and occasionally delerium, catatonia).
- Fever is the predominant feature and malaria must be excluded. Fever coincides with the start of septicaemia, i.e when the organisms are released from the reticuloendothelial system into the blood. It is associated with a relative bradycardia. Pyrexia lasts for 10 days.

Signs occur in week 2 and consist of:
- Erythmatous maculopapular rash that blanches on pressure, giving rise to characteristic rose spots. The rash affects mainly the trunk.
- Splenomegaly occurs in 75% of patients.
- Cervical lymphadenopathy and hepatomegaly are seen in 30%.

Complications arise in week 3 and include:
- Lobar pneumonia.
- Haemolytic anaemia.
- Meningitis.
- Peripheral neuropathy.
- Acute cholecystitis.
- UTI.
- Osteomyelitis.
- Myocarditis.
- GI haemorrhage and perforation due to involvement of the Peyer's patches.
- Diarrhoea usually occurs at week 2.

Carriage:
- Affects 5% and may be associated with persistent infection of the biliary tract.

Investigations show:
- Blood cultures positive in 90% in week 1 and 30% in week 3.
- Leucopenia.
- Positive Widal test occurs at week 2.
- Urine and stool cultures are positive at 2–4 weeks.

The Widal test measures nonspecific antibodies to the somatic O and flagellar H antigens.

Answer 9

D Jaundice is unusual.

Leptospirosis is caused by the spirochaete *Leptospira icterhaemorrhagica*, and is transmitted by contact with infected rat urine.

As the name of the organism suggests, the illness consists crudely of a triad of:
- Jaundice.
- Haemorrhage.
- Renal impairment.

The incubation period is 2–26 days. The Jarisch–Herxheimer reaction (fever, vasodilation, tachycardia) is mediated by the release of an endotoxin, and may rarely complicate treatment.

Tutorial

Symptoms:

- Fever, myalgia, jaundice, and conjunctival hyperaemia are common.
- Bleeding and purpura occur frequently.
- Meningitis – rare, associated with high lymphocyte count and protein in the CSF.
- Renal failure and liver failure are also rare, but are associated with an increased mortality.
- Examination may reveal hepatosplenomegaly and lymphadenopathy.
- The disease is divided into two phases and this will determine which diagnostic test to perform:

– The leptospiraemic phase: Week 1. Bloodcultures will be positive.
– The immune phase: Week 2. Complement fixation is the test of choice.

The organism can be cultured from the urine from 14 days onwards.

Other common features are polymorphonuclear leukocytosis and albuminuria, oliguria, and urinary casts. Treatment is benzylpenicillin 600 mg q.d.s. for 1 week.

Question 10 The following is true for rubella:

A Typically has an incubation period of 7–10 days.
B Is more frequently associated with splenomegaly than is EBV infection.
C Polyarthralgia does not occur.
D Can be prevented by vaccination in >80% of individuals.
E Infection is not hazardous in the first trimester of pregnancy.

Question 11 The following is not a recognized side-effect of griseofulvin:

A Candida.
B Aggravation of SLE.
C Toxic epidermal necrolysis.
D Teratogenicity.
E Peripheral neuropathy.

Question 12 The following is not true of HIV infection:

A Is caused by a retrovirus.
B Seroconversion is usually asymptomatic.
C The antibody against HIV can be detected using ELISA technique.
D Infection is associated with lymphopenia.
E Hypergammaglobulinaemia is a recognized feature.

Answer 10

D Can be prevented by vaccination in >80% of individuals.

Rubella can largely be prevented by vaccination. The infection can affect the foetus in the first trimester and is therefore an indication for termination.

Tutorial

Rubella (German measles) is caused by a spherical RNA virus. The incubation period is 2–3 weeks. Transmission is by droplet spread.

Symptoms:
- Prodrome of fever and myalgia.
- Conjunctivitis.
- Macular rash.

Signs:
- Suboccipital, postauricular, and posterior cervical lymphadenopthy.
- Petechial lesions on palate (Forchheimer spots) are suggestive but not diagnostic.
- Pink macular rash starts at the forehead and spreads downwards. The patient is most infective during this period, and the rash has usually resolved within 2 days.

Complications:
- Secondary bacterial infection.
- Thrombocytopenia and haemorrhage.
- Encephalitis.
- Polyarthralgia which is more common in adults.

Congenital rubella:
- Affects the foetus in the 1st trimester in 70% of cases. Those affected in the 2nd and 3rd are less likely to have congenital abnormalities which include:
- Congenital heart disease (PDA, VSD, coarctation, pulmonary stenosis).
- Ocular (cataracts retinopathy, choroidoretinitis).
- Neurological (sensorineural deafness, mental retardation).
- Microcephaly.
- Renal (renal artery stenosis, polycystic kidneys).

In the expanded rubella syndrome, there are the above features with additional:
- Hepatosplenomegaly.
- Myocarditis.
- Interstitial pneumonia.
- Bony involvement.

Immunization is contraindicated in pregnancy due to the use of a live attenuated virus. Infected mothers should be vaccinated in the post partum period.

Answer 11

A Candida.

Griseofulvin is indicated for the treatment of dermatophyte infections affecting the skin, hair, and nails where topical treatment has failed. It is ineffective in treating yeast infections such as candida. Absorption is improved when it is taken with fatty foods and milk. It can aggravate or precipitate SLE. Males are advised not to father a child within 6 months of treatment due to risks of teratogenicity. Side-effects include headache, nausea, vomiting, photosensitivity, and skin rashes. These include erythema multiforme, toxic epidermal necrolysis, and lupus erythatosis. Agranulocytosis and leucopenia have also been reported.

Answer 12

B Seroconversion is usually asymptomatic.

HIV infection is caused by a retrovirus. It has three main structural genes which are:

- *gag* encodes the nucleocapsid core proteins.
- *pol* codes for major enzymes required for replication (reverse transcriptase, protease, intergrase).
- *env* codes for the outer envelope proteins that enable the virus to enter the cells.

Inside the core of the HIV virus, there are two copies of the RNA genome.

Seroconversion occurs shortly after infection and produces an acute febrile illness resembling infectious mononucleosis or influenza. Infection can be confirmed by detecting the antibody to HIV by ELISA technique.

Lymphopenia is characteristic and is associated with a defect in the T-helper cells, resulting in a marked reduction in cell-mediated immunity.

There are associated B-cell abnormalities, resulting in increased immunoglobulin secretion and hypergammaglobulinaemia.

Question 13 The following is true of infection with *Pneumocystis carinii*:

A Infection is aquired by droplet spread.
B It accounts for 40% of pneumonias seen in HIV infected patients.
C Patients are usually unable to mount a high fever.
D Chest X-ray shows diffuse bilateral interstitial shadowing.
E Nebulized pentamidine is the treatment of choice.

Question 14 In infection with HIV:

A Positive HIV serology on cord blood confirms materno-foetal transmission.
B 30% of patients have circulating lupus anticoagulant.
C Patients respond well to vaccination during early infection.
D There is no association with immune thrombocytopenia purpura.
E There is an association with nasopharyngeal carcinoma.

Question 15 The following is not true of Creutzfeldt–Jakob disease:

A Is transmitted by a slow virus.
B Patients often present with cerebellar ataxia.
C Infection may be transmitted by the use of human growth hormone.
D Brain pathology consists of spongiform change with vacuolation.
E Death occurs within 2 years of onset of symptoms.

Question 16 Recognized complications of falciparum malaria infection do not include:

A Opisthotonos.
B Adult respiratory distress syndrome.
C Hyperlactacidaemia.
D Hyperglycaemia.
E Pulmonary oedema.

Answer 13

D Chest X-ray shows diffuse bilateral interstitial shadowing.

Pneumocystis carinii is a protozoan, which exists as a trophozoite.

Infection is by inhalation and occurs usually during infancy, with reactivation following debility, e.g. severe malnutrition in childhood and HIV in adults. It is responsible for >80% of pneumonia in patients who are HIV-positive.

Tutorial

Symptoms:
- Fever.
- Dry nonproductive cough.
- Tachypnoea.
- Hypoxia (pleurisy and haemoptysis are not features of this illness).
- Physical signs in the chest are minimal or absent.

Diagnosis is made by transbronchial biopsy as the organism cannot be cultured from sputum. Co-trimoxazole is the treatment of choice although nebulized pentamidine may be used alongside.

Infection with PCP is rare in Africans in whom the most common opportunistic infections are TB and cryptococcus.

Answer 14

B 30% of patients have circulating lupus anticoagulant.

All children born to mothers who are HIV-positive are HIV antibody-positive at birth, due to placental passage of maternal IgG.

Specific antibody responses are impaired in early infection and patients do not respond well to vaccination at this time.

In patients with HIV infection the most common cause of thrombocytopenia is ITP. ITP of HIV and also dementia respond to treatment with zidovudine, which is used in symptomatic patients with low CD4 counts. Until recently, CD4 counts and clinical evaluation have been the only predictors of outcome.

HIV is associated with an increased incidence of carcinoma and lymphoma, but is linked more closely to Karposi's sarcoma, whereas EBV is associated with nasopharyngeal and Burkitt's lymphoma.

Other important aspects of the disease include the following:
- Smoking is associated with a poorer prognosis in HIV infection, although the mechanism is unclear.
- Neopterin is a protein released by activated macrophages which predicts the progression of HIV independently of CD4 count. It is not entirely specific in that it is also increased in infections mediated by macrophage activation such as in TB.

Answer 15

B Patients often present with cerebellar ataxia.

Creutzfeldt–Jakob disease is caused by a slow virus, which is particularly resistant to destruction, such that only the high temperature in autoclaves can inactivate it. Although prions are referred to as slow viruses, they consist of a protein particle with no nucleic acid content.

CJD presents with a slowly progressive dementia and myoclonus. Infection with CJD has been contracted using growth hormone from cadaveric pituitary specimens, and can also occur following corneal transplants obtained from post mortem. It is believed that infection can also be transmitted by blood transfusion.

There is a long incubation period of approximately 10 years, and death occurs within 2 years of onset of symptoms.

Tutorial

Other examples of human slow virus infections include:

- Gerstmann–Straussler–Scheinker (GSS) – autosomal dominant, presents with ataxia.
- Kuru – affects the cerebellum causing cerebellar ataxia and dementia. Kuru is spread by tribal funeral practices in Papua New Guinea.
- Subacute sclerosing panencephalitis (SSPE) – caused by the measles virus.
- Progressive multifocal leucoencephalopathy (PML) – caused by papovavirus.
- Progressive rubella panencephalitis (PRP) – caused by rubella virus.

Answer 16

D Hyperglycaemia.

Cerebral falciparum malaria involvement is associated with coma, which may be profound and accompanied by hypertonicity, opisthotonos, posturing of the limbs, hypotonia, and convulsions.

Respiratory ARDS like cerebral involvement is associated with a poor prognosis. Pulmonary oedema is common in patients who have developed renal impairment. Heavy parasitaemia results in sequestration in the tissues and impaired blood flow, resulting in an increase in the serum lactate.

Hypoglycaemia may result from impaired hepatic gluconeogenesis and quinine therapy, and is more common in pregnant women. Severe anaemia, DIC and bleeding, shock, and intravascular haemolysis with haemoglobinuria are all well documented complications.

Question 17 The following is not true of infection with *Mycobacterium leprae*:

A Infection is transmitted to man from infected cattle.
B Lepromatous leprosy is characterized by diffuse thickening of the skin.
C Tuberculoid leprosy is associated with thickening of the nerves.
D Rifampicin is a first line agent for treatment.
E Patients are not infective within weeks of treatment.

Question 18 Typical features of trichiniasis include the following with the exception of:

A Prodromal diarrhoea and vomiting.
B Peri-orbital oedema.
C Vesicular rash.
D Myocarditis is a rare occurrence.
E Tenderness of the muscles.

Question 19 The following is not true for brucellosis:

A Is caused by an intracellular parasite.
B Is acquired from pasteurized milk.
C Is associated with granuloma formation.
D Spinal tenderness may be elicited on examination.
E Tetracycline is an effective treatment.

Answer 17

A Infection is transmitted to man from infected cattle.

Leprosy is a chronic granulomatous disease that is exclusive to humans.

Untreated patients discharge bacilli from the nose, and infection occurs through the nose with local multiplication followed by haematogenous spread to skin and nerve.

Tutorial

Organ involvement:
- Skin: associated with local anaesthesia and loss of sweating.
- Peripheral nerves: nerves are most vulnerable where they lie superficially or in fibrosseous tunnels:
  - Ulnar nerve at the elbow.
  - Median and radial nerves at the wrist.
  - Common peroneal nerve at the knee.
  - Facial nerve as it crosses the zygomatic arch.
  - Eyes – blindness.

Tuberculoid leprosy is associated with:
- Localized symmetrical skin lesions which are hypopigmented.
- Involvement of usually a single peripheral nerve trunk which is enlarged.
- Strongly positive lepromin test.
- Absence of *M. leprae* from the skin.
- Self limiting with good prognosis.

Lepromatous leprosy is associated with:
- Diffuse thickening of the skin, with loss of hair especially the lateral third of the eyebrow.
- Symmetrical sensory neuropathy in glove and stocking distribution.
- Invasion of nasal bridge with collapse.
- Glomerulonephritis.
- Acute orchitis, testicular atrophy, azoospermia, and gynaecomastia.

First line antileprotic drugs are rifampicin, dapsone, and clofazimine.

Newer drugs like clarithromycin, minocycline, and ofloxacin are currently undergoing trials. Within a few days of chemotherapy patients are no longer infective.

Answer 18

C Vesicular rash.

Trichiniasis is caused by the nematode *Trichinella spiralis*. In humans, infection is contracted by eating under-cooked pork. The larval form is also found in cats, dogs, hares, and rats.

Tutorial

Most human infections are asymptomatic. When symptoms do occur, they can be divided into two phases:
- Intestinal – occur in week 1. Symptoms consist of nausea, vomiting, diarrhoea, abdominal pain, and, occasionally, PR bleeding.
- Extra-intestinal – occur in week 2. Larvae encyst in skeletal muscle, causing basophilic degeneration of the muscle fibres and the subsequent development of a hyaline capsule surrounding each larva. Fever, malaise, myalgia, weakness, headache, and peri-orbital oedema can occur. Twenty percent of patients develop a macular or petechial rash. Subconjunctival haemorrhage and splinter haemorrhages may also occur.

Myocarditis is rare and often fatal. CNS involvement leads to seizures, paralysis, coma, and death. Calcification can occur after several months.

Diagnosis is determined from eosinophilia, increased LDH, CK, and serology. Treatment is supportive, with bed rest, salicylates, and corticosteroids in severe infection. Mebendazole and thiabendazole are effective if the diagnosis is made early.

Answer 19

B Is acquired from pasteurized milk.

Brucellosis is caused by *Brucella abortis*, which is an intracellular Gram-negative coccobacillus. It is acquired from cow's milk and is destroyed by pasteurization. The incubation period is 1–3 weeks.

Tutorial

Symptoms:

- Fever, which is typically undulant.
- Lymphadenopathy, hepatomegaly, and spinal tenderness are common.
- The presence of splenomegaly indicates severe infection and also occurs in chronic infection.
- Skeletal complications: arthritis, bursitis, spondylitis, and osteomyelitis.
- Endocarditis, meningo-encephalitis, orchitis, and epididymitis are less common complications.

For diagnosis, blood cultures are positive in 50% of patients. Serology and agglutination tests are of greater value. Tetracycline and co-trimoxazole are the treatments of choice.

Question 20 The following antibiotic is bacteriostatic:

A Nitrofurantoin.
B Tetracyclines.
C Isoniazid.
D Metronidazole.
E Gentamicin.

Question 21 The following is not true of infection with *Helicobacter pylori*:

A Is found in 70% of patients with gastric ulcer.
B Produces urease.
C May be associated with the development of gastric carcinoma.
D Serological tests are most specific to assess cure from infection.
E Does not produce symptoms in most people who are infected.

Question 22 The following is not true of tetanus infection:

A It is caused by a Gram-positive bacillus.
B The incubation period is 3–21 days.
C Trismus is a characteristic early feature.
D The toxin has a predilection for neurones in the anterior horn cells.
E The diagnosis can only be made by isolating the organism and toxin.

Answer 20

B Tetracyclines.

Bactericidal drugs kill bacteria. These drugs are preferable if the host is immunocompromised.

The following are bactericidal:

- Aminoglycosides.
- Cephalosporins.
- Co-trimoxazole.
- Ciprofloxacin.
- Isoniazid.
- Metronidazole.
- Nitrofurantoin.
- Penicillins.
- Rifampicin.

The other drugs are bacteriostatic. They inhibit bacterial replication and rely on host defences to eliminate the bacteria. Bactericidal drugs in combination are synergistic. The combination of a bactericidal drug with a bacteriostatic drug results in antagonism.

Answer 21

D Serological tests are most specific to assess cure from infection.

Helicobacter pylori is a Gram-negative bacterium found in 70% of patients with gastric ulcers, and in 90% of patients with duodenal ulcers. It is also found in 50% of the population over the age of 50 years.

The bacteria produce urease, which forms the basis of the breath test used to diagnose infection. Urease is an enzyme which hydrolyzes urea to form ammonia and CO_2. In patients who have been treated for *H. pylori* infection, a breath test should not be performed until 28 days after tratment is completed.

H. pylori is classified as a class I carcinogen by the WHO, and some studies have suggested a definite link with gastric carcinoma. Eradicating infection reduces ulcer relapse but whether it reduces the risk of neoplasia is not known. Only a minority of patients who are infected develop symptoms.

Answer 22

E The diagnosis can only be made by isolating the organism and toxin.

Tetanus is caused by a Gram-positive, anaerobic, spore-forming bacillus found in soil and intestinal flora of man and animals. The incubation period is 3–21 days but may rarely occur several years after the original injury.

Infection is caused by a potent protein neurotoxin which has a high affinity for the presynaptic terminals of the inhibitory spinal neurones in the anterior horn and spinal cord. At these terminals the release of inhibitory neurotransmitters is prevented, resulting in unopposed and excessive activity of the alpha motor neurones.

The diagnosis is clinical but supporting microbiological evidence is occasionally possible.

9 Neurology

Question 1 IIIrd nerve palsy is unlikely to occur in:

A Motor neurone disease.
B Neurosyphilis.
C Temporal arteritis.
D Intracranial aneurysm.
E Diabetes mellitus.

Question 2 The following is not a feature of the VII nerve:

A Origin occurs from a nucleus at the pons.
B Lesion at the cerebellopontine angle is associated with impaired facial sensation.
C Supplies the muscles of mastication.
D Supplies taste to the anterior two-thirds of the tongue.
E An upper motor neurone lesion spares the forehead on the contralateral side.

Question 3 The following is true of trigeminal neuralgia:

A Spontaneous remission may occur.
B There is loss of sensation on the affected side of the face.
C It is frequently bilateral.
D Is relieved by carbimazole.
E The corneal reflex on the affected side is absent.

Question 4 The pupillary light reflex is independent of the integrity of:

A Occipital cortex.
B Optic nerve.
C Edinger–Westphal nucleus.
D Ciliary ganglion.
E Lateral geniculate body.

Answer 1

A Motor neurone disease.

Aneurysm of the posterior communicating artery causes a painful IIIrd nerve palsy. Aneurysms of the internal carotids and cavernous sinus can also produce a IIIrd nerve palsy. Other causes of IIIrd nerve palsy include:
- Diabetes mellitus.
- Atherosclerosis.
- Temporal arteritis.
- Multiple sclerosis.
- Sarcoidosis.
- Herpes zoster.
- Cholesteatoma.
- Myasthenia gravis.
- Neurosyphilis.
- Brainstem vascular lesions (Weber's syndrome).
- Midbrain infarction.
- Increased ICP (pressure from the uncus of the temporal lobe as it herniates through the tentorium).

Motor neurone disease principally affects the bulbar nerves (progressive bulbar palsy), while the ocular nerves are spared. This results in symptoms of dysarthria, dysphagia, nasal regurgitation, and choking. Signs include a spastic weak palate and a wasted fibrillating tongue.

Acoustic neuroma at the cerebellopontine angle affects:
- Vth nerve: resulting in facial numbness and absent corneal reflex.
- VIIth nerve: resulting in facial weakness.
- VIIIth nerve: resulting in deafness and vertigo.

Symptoms may be progressive as the neuroma enlarges and may be accompanied by cerebellar ataxia.

Tutorial

Signs of IIIrd nerve palsy:
- Unilateral ptosis.
- Fixed dilated pupil.
- Divergent strabismus.
- Difficulty in looking upwards or focussing on near objects.

'Sparing of the pupil' may occur by parasympathetic fibres that run discretely on the surface of the IIIrd nerve, in which case the pupil will react normally. In diabetes, infarction usually spares the pupil. The patient will still be able to abduct the eye (VIth nerve) and intort the eye (IVth nerve).

Answer 2

C Supplies the muscles of mastication.

The facial (VIIth) nerve arises from a nucleus at the tegmentum of the pons. At close proximity to its origin, it encircles the VIth nerve nucleus and the parapontine reticular formation. Lesions at the pons level include:
- Pontine tumours, e.g. gliomas.
- Vascular accidents.
- Demyelination.

Signs at this level include:
- UMN VIIth nerve weakness.
- Failure of conjugate gaze.
- Contralateral hemiparesis.
- Drowsiness.

Lesions at the cerebellopontine angle, e.g. acoustic neuroma, meningioma affect the Vth, VIth, and VIIIth nerves, resulting in:
- Facial weakness.
- Impaired facial sensation.
- Deafness and vertigo.

Lesions at the petrous part of the temporal bone cause:
- Loss of taste at the anterior two-thirds of the tongue.
- Hyperacusis due to paralysis of the stapedius muscle.

The facial nerve is a motor nerve supplying all muscles of facial expression. The muscles of mastication are supplied by the trigeminal nerve.

Tutorial

Causes of bilateral LMN facial nerve palsy:
- Guillain–Barré syndrome.
- Motor neurone disease.
- Poliomyelitis.
- Post-meningitis.
- Bilateral acoustic neuromas.
- Sarcoidosis.
- Infectious mononucleosis.
- Lepromatous leprosy.
- Tetanus.
- Congenital (Moebius syndrome).

Answer 3

A Spontaneous remission may occur.

Trigeminal neuralgia occurs almost always in the elderly. Younger patients who develop the condition under the age of 50 years should be investigated for multiple sclerosis and underlying tumour. Symptoms include paroxysms of sharp stabbing pain in the distribution of the Vth nerve unilaterally.

The pain characteristically starts in the mandibular division and spreads to the maxillary division. The ophthalmic division is rarely involved. Paroxysms are stereotyped in that they are brought on by stimulation of a specific trigger zone on the face, e.g. the lips or the side of the nose whilst eating, shaving, or as a result of exposure to cold winds. The pain characteristically does not occur at night. Spontaneous remissions may last for years. Trigeminal nerve function is preserved with no loss of facial sensation or corneal reflex.

Carbamazepine is the treatment of choice but phenytoin is also effective. Occasionally symptoms may be caused by an aberrant blood vessel overlying the nerve or ganglion and dissection completely resolves the symptoms. (Note: there is a definite suicide risk.)

Answer 4

A Occipital cortex.

When light is shone into the eye the following sequence of events occurs:

- Afferent pathway: afferent fibres pass in the optic nerves down the optic tracts with some crossover in the chiasm to both lateral geniculate bodies, and relay to the Edinger–Westphal nucleus of the IIIrd nerve.
- Efferent pathway: parasympathetic fibres pass from each Edinger–Westphal nucleus via the oculomotor nerve to the ciliary ganglion, and then to the pupil.

The cortex is not involved. Convergence originates from the cortex and is relayed to the pupil via the IIIrd nerve nuclei. The optic nerve, tract, and lateral geniculate bodies are not involved.

Question 5 A small pupil is not a feature of:

A Acute retrobulbar neuritis.
B Horner's syndrome.
C Tabes dorsalis.
D Pontine lesions.
E Diabetes.

Question 6 Unilateral ptosis is most likely to be seen in:

A Dystrophia myotonica.
B Migranous neuralgia.
C Congenital Horner's syndrome.
D Syringobulbia.
E Cavernous sinus thrombosis.

Question 7 Absent knee jerks and extensor plantars are not a feature of:

A Taboparesis.
B Friedreich's ataxia.
C Motor neurone disease.
D Multiple sclerosis.
E B12 deficiency.

Answer 5

A Acute retrobulbar neuritis.

In tabes dorsalis, the pupil is:
- Constricted.
- Irregular.
- The direct light reflex is absent.
- The convergence reflex is intact.

In Horner's syndrome there is unilateral:
- Ptosis.
- Constricted pupil with normal reactions.
- Anhidrosis (reduced sweating over face).
- Enophthalmos (indrawing of the orbital contents).

The lesion in Horner's sundrome may be central, preganglionic, or post-ganglionic. Hydroxyamphetamine drops release noradrenaline from the terminal axons if they are intact, and hence will dilate the pupil in central and preganglionic Horner's syndrome. Phenylephrine dilates the normal and abnormal pupil equally in central and preganglionic lesions. In the case of post-ganglionic lesions, there is denervation hypersensitivity causing the pupil to dilate more widely. Cocaine dilates the normal eye only.

In acute retrobulbar neuritis the pupil is dilated. Holmes–Adie (myotonic) pupil is caused by denervation of the ciliary ganglion. The condition is more common in women and is usually unilateral. The pupil is dilated and responds sluggishly to light with incomplete constriction. The pupil can be made to respond briskly by the addition of 25% metacholine eye drops. It is associated with diminished or absent tendon reflexes and is of no pathological significance.

Other causes of constricted pupils:
- Pontine haemorrhage.
- Senile miosis.
- Drugs, e.g. pilocarpine, opiates.

Answer 6

A Dystrophia myotonica.

Horner's syndrome is a well recognized cause of unilateral ptosis and may be caused by:
- Damage to the sympathetic pathways to the medulla as in syringobulbia.
- Lesions to the first thoracic root in the thoracic outlet syndrome.
- External carotid artery dilatation as in migranous neuralgia.

The occulomotor nerve runs in the lateral wall of the cavernous sinus and can be damaged in cavernous sinus thrombosis causing a unilateral ptosis. Congenital ptosis can be unilateral. Isolated facial nerve palsy does not cause ptosis.

Ptosis is usually bilateral in:
- Dystrophia myotonica – an autosomal dominant disease, associated with progressive weakness of the distal muscles.
- Facio-scapulo-humeral dystrophy.
- Taboparesis.
- Myasthenia gravis.

Answer 7

D Multiple sclerosis.

Absent reflexes imply a LMN lesion and extensor planters a UMN lesion.

Absent knee jerks and extensor planters are seen in:
- Taboparesis.
- Motor neurone disease.
- Subacute combined degeneration of the cord.
- Friedreich's ataxia.
- Conus medullaris.
- B12 deficiency.
- Spinal cord compression at the 4th lumbar level.
- Spinal shock.
- Diabetic amyotrophy.

Cervical spondylosis is associated with UMN signs. Multiple sclerosis commonly involves the corticospinal tracts leading to hyper-reflexia and extensor plantar responses. Peroneal muscular atrophy results in absent ankle jerks but normal or absent plantar responses.

Question 8 Muscle fasciculation is not a feature of:

A Motor neurone disease.
B Cervical spondylosis.
C Friedreich's ataxia.
D Syringomyelia.
E Neuralgic amyotrophy.

Question 9 Spastic paraplegia complicates all except:

A B12 deficiency.
B Chronic lead poisoning.
C Hodgkin's disease.
D Paget's disease.
E Neurofibromatosis.

Question 10 A reduced CSF glucose is seen in:

A Sarcoidosis.
B Motor neurone disease.
C Multiple sclerosis.
D Tuberculous meningitis.
E Spinal cord compression.

Question 11 An elevated CSF protein is not a feature of:

A Bacterial meningitis.
B Sarcoidosis.
C Subarachnoid haemorrhage.
D Motor neurone disease.
E Multiple sclerosis.

Answer 8

C Friedreich's ataxia.

Muscle fasciculations are a feature of lower motor neurone lesions. They consist of irregular contractions of muscle fibres which are innervated by the same motor unit. Causes of muscle fasciculations are:

- Anterior horn cell disease:
  - Motor neurone disease.
  - Acute poliomyelitis.
  - Spinal root damage.
  - Cervical spondylosis.
  - Lumbar canal stenosis.
  - Neuralgic amyotrophy.
- Cranial or peripheral nerve damage:
  - Trauma.
  - Compression.
  - Polyneuropathy.
- Drugs and metabolic disorders:
  - Thyrotoxicosis.
  - Hyponatraemia.
  - Hypomagnesaemia.
  - Lithium.
  - Anticholinesterases.

Other features of lower motor neurone lesions:

- Muscle weakness.
- Wasting.
- Hypotonia.
- Absent reflexes.
- Muscle contractures.
- Trophic changes in skin and nails.

Answer 9

B Chronic lead poisoning.

Spastic paraparesis is caused by anything that produces cord compression. Causes include:

Extradural compression (disorders of the vertebrae) (45%):

- Cervical spondylosis.
- Vertebral collapse (myeloma, carcinoma, osteoporosis).
- Tuberculosis.
- Paget's disease.
- Cervical and lumbar canal stenosis.
- Abscess.
- Prolapsed intervertebral disc.

Intradural compression (meningeal disorders) (45%):

- Neurofibroma (dumb-bell tumours).
- Meningioma (usually thoracic and more common in women).

Intramedullary (lesions of the spinal cord) (5–10%):

- Gliomas.
- Ependymomas.

Other causes:

- Multiple sclerosis.
- SACD of the cord.
- Parasagittal meningioma.
- Transverse myelitis.
- Anterior spinal artery thrombosis.
- Motor neurone disease.
- B12 deficiency.

Signs of spastic paraparesis:

- UMN weakness of the lower limbs (with increased tone, exaggerated tendon reflexes).
- Loss of sphincter control (indicative of poor prognosis).
- Loss of abdominal reflexes (if the lesion is in or above the thoracic cord).

Answer 10

D Tuberculous meningitis.

A low CSF glucose is seen in active infection and also in conditions where there are more cells (usually blood cells) around the meninges. Causes include:

Infections:

- Bacterial meningitis.
- TB meningitis.
- Unusual in viral meningitis but is seen in mumps meningitis.
- Fungal, cryptococcal, amoebic meningitis.
- CNS cysticercosis.

Other:

- SAH.
- CNS vasculitis.

Answer 11

E Multiple sclerosis.

In multiple sclerosis, the CSF protein is normal but the gamma globulin fraction is elevated.

Tutorial

Causes of increased CSF protein include:

Infection:
- TB, bacterial, viral, and fungal meningitis.
- Leptospirosis, amoebic meningo-encephalitis, viral encephalitis.
- Cerebral abscess.
- Neurosyphilis.

Granulomatous disease:
- Sarcoidosis.

Cerebrovascular accidents:
- Embolism, infarction.
- Subdural haematoma.

Cerebral malignancy.
Cord compression.
Motor neurone disease.

Endocrine:
- Hypothyroidism.
- Diabetes mellitus.

Causes of very high CSF protein:
- Acoustic neuroma.
- Guillain–Barré syndrome.
- Froin's syndrome (spinal block due to epidural abscess or tumour).

Question 12 Idiopathic intracranial hypertension:

A Is more common in women with psychiatric disorders.
B Presents with episodic altered consciousness.
C CT scan of the brain is abnormal.
D The condition may complicate therapy with tetracyclines.
E Treatment is with regular venesection.

Question 13 Features of motor neurone disease include:

A Ptosis.
B Sensory neuropathy.
C Impaired joint position.
D Wasting of the small muscles of the hands.
E Nystagmus.

Answer 12

D The condition may complicate therapy with tetracyclines.

Idiopathic intracranial hypertension affects mainly young overweight women who often have menstrual problems. It presents most commonly with visual problems as a result of papilloedema caused by increased ICP. There may be false localizing signs of increased ICP, e.g. VIth nerve palsy, and in severe untreated cases, blindness due to infarction of the optic nerve. CT brain scan is normal, i.e. no hydrocephalus.

In most cases no cause can be found. The following, however, are recognized causes:

- Oral contraceptive pill.
- Pregnancy.
- Hypoparathyroidism.
- Addison's disease.
- Vitamin A toxicity and deficiency.
- Tetracycline toxicity.

Treatment includes weight loss, repeated lumbar puncture, and thiaizide diuretics to reduce ICP. In resistant cases where vision is at risk, surgical decompression and shunting may be necessary.

Answer 13

D Wasting of the small muscles of the hands.

Motor neurone disease is a sporadic disease of unknown cause. It is more common in men and affects the motor neurones as a result of degeneration of the:

- Betz cells.
- Pyramidal fibres.
- Cranial nerve nuclei.
- Anterior horn cells.

Both upper and lower motor neurones may be affected but there is never any sensory neuropathy, which distinguishes it from multiple sclerosis and polyneuropathies.

It never affects the external ocular muscles which are supplied by nerves III, IV, and VI, hence ptosis is not a feature. There are never any cerebellar or extrapyramidal signs. Dementia is unusual with awareness being preserved. Sphincter disturbance may occur late in the disease but is rare. It is always fatal within 3–5 years of diagnosis.

Tutorial

Syndromes of motor neurone disease:

Progressive muscular atrophy:

- Occurs in 25% of patients.
- Is caused by degeneration of the anterior horn cells.
- Characterized by small muscle wasting affecting the distal muscles before the proximal ones.
- Better prognosis than AML.

Signs:

- Wasting of small muscles of hand progressing to forearm.
- Weakness.
- Fasciculation is common.
- Tendon reflexes are usually absent but may be preserved or exaggerated, due to loss of motor neurones at the corticospinal tracts.

Amyotrophic lateral sclerosis:

- Affects 50% of patients.
- Caused by degeneration of the corticospinal tracts.

Signs:

- LMN wasting.
- UMN hyper-reflexia.
- Weakness.
- Progressive spastic tetra or paraparesis.

Progressive bulbar palsy:

- Affects 25% of patients.
- Due to degeneration of lower cranial nerve nuclei.
- More common in women.

Signs:

- Dysarthria.
- Dysphagia.
- Nasal regurgitation of fluids.
- Choking.
- Wasted fibrillating tongue.
- Spastic weak palate.

Question 14 Choreiform movements do not occur in:

A Huntington's disease.
B Therapy with levodopa.
C Thyrotoxicosis.
D Treatment with phenothiazines.
E Polycythaemia vera.

Question 15 Wasting of the small muscles of the hand is not a feature of:

A Syringomyelia.
B Friedreich's ataxia.
C Cervical myelopathy.
D Motor neurone disease.
E Meningovascular syphilis.

Question 16 The following is not associated with the development of extrapyramidal rigidity:

A Carbon monoxide poisoning.
B Lead poisoning.
C Phenothiazine therapy.
D Smoking.
E Wilson's disease.

Answer 14

D Treatment with phenothiazines.

Chorea is a dyskinesia consisting of jerky, semi purposeful, and sometimes explosive movements following each other and flitting from one part of the body to the next.

Causes of chorea:
- Huntington's disease.
- Benign hereditary chorea.
- Pregnancy.
- Drugs:
  - Alcohol.
  - Phenytoin.
  - Levodopa.
  - OCP.
- Infections:
  - Encephalitis lethargica.
  - Sydnenham's chorea.
  - SLE.
- Thyrotoxicosis.
- Polycythaemia vera.
- CVA:
  - Thrombosis/ haemorrhage.
  - Subdural haematoma.
  - Intracranial tumour.

Tutorial

Huntington's chorea
This is autosomal dominant, with complete penetrance. Onset is usually between 5th and 6th decades with progressive chorea and dementia. There is associated personality change with increased irritability. Epilepsy is common. Younger patients may have marked extrapyramidal rigidity and have usually inherited the disease from their father.

Incidence: 1/20 000; children have 50% likelihood of being affected.

Gene: G8 locus of chromosome 4.

Pathology
- Cerebral atrophy with loss of small neurones in the caudate nucleus and putamen.
- Changes in neurotransmitters: reduction in enzymes producing acetylcholine and GABA in the striatum; depletion of GABA and ACE in the subtantia nigra; increased somatostatin in the corpus striatum.

In contrast to Parkinson's disease, dopamine and tyrosine hydroxylase activity are normal. Tetrabenazine can be used to control the chorea, phenothiazines and butyrophenones can be used for sedation in hyperkinetic patients.

Sydenham's chorea
Chorea is associated with rheumatic fever but occurs in <50% of patients 3 months after infection. It is a transient chorea of adolescence and childhood and can recur later in life during pregnancy (chorea gravidarum), or in patients on OCP. There is a diffuse encephalitis.

Temperature and ESR are usually, but not always, normal.

Answer 15

B Friedreich's ataxia.

Cord lesions at T1 level occur in syringomyelia causing wasting of the small muscles of the hand. Other recognized causes of such cord lesions include motor neurone disease, meningovascular syphilis, and compression by tumour.

Root lesions occurring in cervical spondylosis also cause muscle wasting. Brachial plexus lesions, e.g. Klumpke's paralysis, cervical rib, and ulnar or median nerve lesions also cause small muscle wasting in the hands.

Answer 16

D Smoking.

Extrapyramidal rigidity can be caused by a number of drugs and poisons.

Carbon monoxide poisoning is a well documented cause of Parkinson's disease, following chronic exposure. Acute toxicity is associated with headache, nausea, vomiting, cognitive impairment, coma, and a classical pink colouration of the skin. This is treated with high concentration oxygen.

Drugs:
- Phenothiazines, reserpine, butyrophenones: induce a syndrome with rigidity and slowness but little tremor.
- Methyldopa, tricyclic antidepressants: cause some slowing of movement.

  In iatrogenic causes the syndrome does not progress and disappears when the drug is stopped. These cases do not respond to levodopa.
- MPTP (1-methyl 4-phenyl 1,2,5,6-tetrahydropyridine): causes irreversible Parkinson's disease following ingestion of minute amounts. The effects are seen as a result of synthetic opiate manufacture by drug addicts in California in 1982.

Other causes of Parkinson's disease:
- Malignant neuroleptic syndrome (malignant pyrexia, extrapyramidal rigidity, autonomic disturbance).
- Wilson's disease (deposition of copper in the basal ganglia).
- Arteriosclerosis.
- Encephalitis lethargica.
- Communicating hydrocephalus.
- Lead poisoning is associated with mental retardation, abdominal pain, and constipation. There may be an associated peripheral neuropathy causing wrist and foot drop. Toxicity may lead to encephalopathy, seizures, and coma. Dense metaphyseal bands (lead lines) are seen at the end of long bones and blue lines on the gums. There is a macrocytic anaemia with basophilic stippling. Treatment is with sodium EDTA although D-penicillamine and dimercaprol have also been used.
- Parkinson-plus syndromes (supranuclear palsy).
- Steel–Richardson–Olszewski syndrome: dementia, absent vertical gaze.
- Shy–Drager syndrome: atonic bladder, orthostatic hypotension.

Question 17 Absence seizures are associated with:

A Wandering.
B Olfactory aura.
C Visual hallucinations.
D Spike wave changes at 3 Hz on EEG.
E *Déjà vu* experience.

Question 18 The following is not a feature of neurofibromatosis:

A Optic atrophy.
B Pigmentation.
C Paroxysms of hypertension.
D Conductive deafness.
E Nonlymphocytic leukaemia.

Question 19 The following is not a characteristic finding in Duchenne muscular dystrophy:

A Wasting of the small muscles of the hands.
B Increased serum creatinine kinase.
C X-linked inheritance.
D Pseudohypertrophy of the muscles.
E Myopathic pattern on EMG.

Answer 17

D Spike wave changes at 3 Hz on EEG.

The rest are features of temporal lobe epilepsy which manifests as a complex partial seizure associated with episodes of impaired consciousness, often with olfactory aura followed by automatism. There may be feelings of unreality (*jamais vu*) or overfamiliarity (*déjà vu*). Visual hallucinations may occur.

Symptoms may be accompanied by absence attacks or vertigo.

Answer 18

D Conductive deafness.

Neurofibromatosis is an autosomal dominant neurocutaneous disorder which has many associations.

Typical features:
- Cutaneous neurofibromas.
- Plexiform neurones.
- 5+ *café-au-lait* spots.
- Axillary freckling.

Increased tendency towards:
- Bilateral acoustic neuromas (deafness).
- Phaeochromocytoma (sustained and paroxysmal hypertension).
- Cerebral astrocytomas (optic gliomas).
- Meningioma.
- Scoliosis.
- Renal artery stenosis.
- Pulmonary fibrosis.
- Hypertrophic cardiomyopathy.
- Local gigantism of a limb.
- Wilm's tumour.
- Fibrous dysplasia of bone.
- Nonlymphocytic leukaemia.

Answer 19

A Wasting of the small muscles of the hands.

DMD is a sex linked recessive condition almost exclusive to males.

The gene is on the short arm of the X chromosome (Xp21) and 30% of cases are sporadic. The condition presents in early childhood at around 4 years with clumsy walking and difficulty standing upright. Patients can be seen to use their arms to climb up their legs (Gower's sign). The proximal limbs are affected first with onset of weakness and associated pseudohypertrophy of the calves. The myocardium is also affected.

Most patients are disabled by the age of 10 years and die by the age of 20 years.

Investigations show:
- Raised CK (fourfold).
- Muscle biopsy variation in fibre size with necrosis and fatty infiltration.
- EMG shows a myopathic pattern.

Carrier females show increased CK in 70% of cases and 30% have abnormal EMG and muscle biopsy.

Question 20 The following statement is not true:

A A grasp reflex may result from a lesion in the frontal lobe.
B Nystagmus is seen in lesions of the occipital cortex.
C The jaw jerk is absent in bulbar palsy.
D The palatal gag reflex is absent in bulbar palsy.
E Parietal lobe disease may be associated with lower quadrantanopia.

Question 21 The following statement is not true regarding lateral medullary syndrome:

A May be caused by thrombo-embolism of the vertebral artery.
B Is associated with ipsilateral palatal paralysis.
C There is ipsilateral ataxia of the limbs.
D There is ipsilateral loss of pain and temperature sensation in the face.
E There is a contralateral Horner's syndrome.

Question 22 The following is not a recognized cause of cerebral calcification:

A Tuberous sclerosis.
B Congenital toxoplasmosis.
C Sturge–Weber syndrome.
D Paget's disease.
E Pseudohypoparathyroidism.

Answer 20

B Nystagmus is seen in lesions of the occipital cortex.

Nystagmus is seen in parietal lobe lesions and in such circumstances may be accompanied by asterognosis, finger agnosia, sensory inattention, dressing apraxia, prosopagnosia, and ideomotor apraxia. It may manifest as defect of attention in the contralateral visual field and produce a lower quadrantonopic visual field defect.

The jaw jerk is exaggerated in pseudobulbar palsy and is absent by definition in bulbar palsy.

Answer 21

E There is a contralateral Horner's syndrome.

The lateral medullary syndrome is the commonest brainstem vascular syndrome. It is caused by thrombosis of the posterior inferior cerebellar artery or the vertebral artery. It presents acutely with:
- Vertigo.
- Vomiting.
- Hiccoughs.
- Ipsilateral facial pain.
- Dysphagia and dysarthria may occur.

Ipsilateral:
- Palatal paralysis.
- Horner's syndrome.
- Spinothalamic sensory loss in the face.
- Cerebellar signs in the limbs, i.e. ataxia.

Contralateral:
- Spinothalamic loss in the body, i.e. loss of pain and temperature.

Answer 22

D Paget's disease.

Tutorial

Other important causes of intracerebral calcification include:
- Congenital toxoplasmosis.
- Craniopharyngioma (suprasellar calcification).
- Chronic subdural haematoma.
- TB.
- Cysticercosis.
- Normal pineal gland.

Intracerebral calcification occurs in:
- Tuberose sclerosis: an autosomal dominant condition consisting of a triad of adenoma sebaceum (angiofibromas around the nose), epilepsy, and mental retardation.
- Sturge–Weber syndrome: a unilateral port wine stain occurs, most frequently seen in the ophthalmic division of the trigeminal nerve. There are associated leptimeningeal angioma usually in the parieto-occipital region, which calcify.
- Calcification of the basal ganglia is seen in hyperparathyroidism and pseudohyperparathyroidism.
- Acute abscesses do not calcify although healed old abscesses may show calcification.

Question 23 Claw feet deformities are seen in all except:

A Charcot's arthropathy.
B Tabes dorsalis.
C Syringomyelia.
D Friedreich's ataxia.
E Peroneal muscular atrophy.

Question 24 The following are predictors of a poor outcome following a head injury except:

A Hypertension.
B Prolonged duration of coma.
C Post-traumatic amnesia lasting 72 hours.
D Mild hypothermia.
E Skull fracture.

Question 25 In a right-sided internuclear ophthalmoplegia:

A The lesion is in the left median longitudinal fasciculus.
B On attempted left lateral gaze, the right eye fails to adduct.
C The right eye develops coarse nystagmus on adduction.
D A past medical history of optic neuritis is not significant.
E Is caused by pathology in the cerebral cortex.

Answer 23

A Charcot's arthropathy.

Clawing of the foot occurs in:
- Syringomyelia: shoulder most commonly affected with dissociated sensory loss.
- Diabetes mellitus: joints of the foot are principally affected with evidence of peripheral neuropathy.
- Tabes dorsalis: knee and ankle involvement.
- Leprosy: any joint.
- Lateral popliteal nerve palsy causes foot drop.
- Friedreich's ataxia.
- Peroneal atrophy.

Charcots joints are swollen, unstable, and grossly deformed joints. They are not associated with clawing of the foot.

Answer 24

D Mild hypothermia.

General factors indicating a bad prognosis following a head injury include:
- Hypertension.
- Fever >39°C (102°F).
- Advancing age.

Neurological predictors of poor outcome include:
- Prolonged coma or post-traumatic amnesia lasting >24 hours.
- Skull fracture, which may be complicated by extra-dural haematoma due to laceration of the meningeal artery, subdural haematoma, and CSF rhinorrhoea caused by dural tears increasing the possibility of meningitis.
- Decerebrate rigidity.
- Extensor spasms.

Answer 25

B On attempted left lateral gaze, the right eye fails to adduct.

In a right internucleur ophthalmoplegia, the lesion is in the right median longitudinal fasciculus. On attempted left lateral gaze, the right eye fails to adduct and the left eye develops a coarse nystagmus.

Multiple sclerosis is an important cause and a past history of optic neuritis is of great significance because of this. A single episode of INO is not diagnostic for MS, nor is the finding of oligoclonal bands in the CSF. Bilateral INO is, however, diagnostic for MS. The pathology is in the brainstem.

INO may also occur in myasthenia gravis, and oligoclonal bands are also seen in other inflammatory lesions, e.g. sarcoidosis.

10 Psychiatry

Question 1 The following complaint is not commonly psychogenic:

A Exhaustion.
B Impotence.
C Inability to take a deep enough breath.
D Left inframammary pain.
E Seeing coloured halos around lights.

Question 2 The following is not true for anorexia nervosa:

A Occurs more frequently in higher socio-economic groups.
B May include episodes of over eating.
C May present with menstrual abnormalities.
D Does not occur before puberty.
E Is rarely recognized by the patient as an illness.

Question 3 A female aged 50 years becomes depressed. The following feature suggests that the response to tricyclic antidepressants is not likely to be effective:

A Psychomotor retardation.
B Complaints of lack of motivation.
C Auditory hallucinations.
D Stable premorbid personality.
E Diurnal variation in severity of depression.

Question 4 The following statement about Alzheimer's disease is not correct:

A Its neuropathology is indistinguishable from that of senile dementia.
B There is an increased incidence of the disorder in first degree relatives.
C There are characteristic changes in the CSF.
D On CT scanning there is often generalized atrophy particularly of the cerebral cortex.
E It may be mimicked by depressive illness.

Question 5 Insomnia is not a characteristic feature of:

A Mania.
B Conversion hysteria.
C Depressive illness.
D Delirium tremens.
E Treatment with beta-blockers.

Answer 1

E Seeing coloured halos around lights.

The following symptoms are often psychogenic in origin:
- Exhaustion.
- Impotence.
- Inability to take a deep enough breath.
- Left inframammary pain.

Individual neurotic symptoms are very common in the general population and may be evident in up to 80% of adults. On their own, such symptoms do not warrant a psychiatric diagnosis.

Answer 2

D Does not occur before puberty.

High risk groups include members from higher socio-economic groups, models, dancers, and nurses. One in three patients indulge in periodic binges of high carbohydrate foods usually followed by self-induced vomiting or purgation. The condition usually begins in the teens and early 20s.

The degree of depression is less than might be expected considering the degree of emaciation and disruption of family life. Most patients are optimistic and deny any seriousness of the condition. For this reason, few patients agree to treatment.

Answer 3

C Auditory hallucinations.

Symptoms of endogenous depression respond well. These are low moods, early morning wakening, low self-esteem, loss of interest in everyday events, reduced libido, constipation, and psychomotor retardation.

Auditory hallucinations and paranoid delusions are features of psychotic depression. In psychotic depression, patients often have auditory hallucinations where they hear voices telling them to commit suicide and saying derogatory things about them.

Answer 4

C There are characteristic changes in the CSF.

Senile dementia of the Alzheimer's type (SDAT) is the most common cause of dementia in old age. Historically, senile dementia has been distinguished from Alzheimer's, which is the most common cause of dementia before the age of 65 years. The latter is still much less common than SDAT. However, the two conditions show very similar brain pathology.

First degree relatives of sufferers are four times more likely to develop the disease than the general population. Pathologically there is generalized atrophy of the brain, especially the cerebral cortex.

There may be some confusion on initial presentation, as symptoms such as impaired concentration can also suggest a possible depressive illness.

Histologically:
- There is severe nerve cell loss with marked gliosis.
- Extracellular senile plaques (abnormal neuronal processes intermingled with astrocytes and microglia, larger plaques may contain amyloid).
- Intraneuronal neurofibrillary tangles (aggregated bundles of filaments within the perikaryon of pyramidal neurones).

Answer 5

B Conversion hysteria.

In mania and delirium tremens sleep is commonly disturbed. Insomnia and early morning wakening can be an early sign of a manic episode. Patients with endogenous depression have characteristic early morning wakening but can also suffer from insomnia. Sleep is not affected in conversion hysteria.

Tutorial

Types of insomnia

There are two broad categories:
- Chronic insomnia – lasting for several weeks, months, or even years.
- Transient insomnia – lasting for a few nights or weeks only, usually connected to a stressful event, e.g. an exam, a bereavement.

Main causes

Insomnia is a condition that is caused by something else! Sometimes it will not be immediately obvious what the causes are, but the following list might give clues:

- States of mind – anxiety, depression, worry, anger, grief, anticipating a difficult event.
- Change – moving house/city, starting university.
- Environment – noise, discomfort, time zone change.
- Pain – one of the commonest causes.
- Medical conditions – heart, breathing, stomach, digestive, high blood pressure, arthritis, anorexia.
- Recreational drugs – including nicotine, caffeine, heroin, cocaine, amphetamines, LSD, cannabis.
- Sleeping pills and tranquillisers – can actually cause sleep disturbance.
- Other prescription drugs – including some contraceptives, diuretics, slimming pills, beta-blockers, stimulants.

Mania:

- Hallmark: infectious optimism, euphoria (some patients are hostile and aggressive).
- Mood is usually changeable.
- Hallucinations occur in 10% and are always auditory.
- Formal thought disorder: flight of ideas accompanied by pressure of speech.
- Sexual activity and interest are increased.

Question 6 The following is true for nocturnal enuresis:

A Is often associated with a reduction in day frequency.
B Can often be helped by restriction of fluid intake before bedtime.
C Is usually associated with urinary tract infection.
D May be associated with behaviour disturbance.
E Is usually helped by administration of phenobarbitone.

Question 7 The following is not a common feature of anxiety:

A Palpitations.
B Epigastric discomfort.
C Constipation.
D Difficulty with breathing.
E Sweating.

Question 8 The following is not likely to be found in a patient suffering from amnesic Korsakoff's syndrome:

A Tachycardia.
B Confabulation.
C Peripheral neuropathy.
D Clouding of consciousness.
E Sweating.

Question 9 That a psychosis is schizophrenic rather than depressive is suggested by all except the following:

A Delusions of grandeur.
B Hopelessness.
C Delusions of passivity.
D Thought blocking.
E Aggressive behaviour.

Answer 6

D May be associated with behaviour disturbance.

Patients with nocturnal enuresis often have day frequency and suffer from bedwetting even if fluids are restricted at night. It is a diagnosis of exclusion such that UTI, glycosuria, and bladder abnormalities have been investigated for and excluded prior to the diagnosis being made.

Enuresis may occur as part of a conduct disorder of the antisocial type.

Treatment is with behaviour techniques for best results, but tricyclic antidepressants are also used.

Tutorial

Enuresis:
- Affects 10% of 10 year olds and 1% of 18 year olds.
- It is more common in boys.
- It is more common in larger families and other types of social adversity, like family discord or institutional upbringing.
- There is also a genetic component with a positive family history in first degree relatives in the majority of cases.

Answer 7

C Constipation.

Anxiety is associated with palpitations, difficulty with breathing, sweating, and loose motions or frank diarrhoea.

Answer 8

D Clouding of consciousness.

Lesions at the hypothalamic diencephalic region give rise to the clinical picture of Korsakoff's psychosis. This is characterized by impairment of memory (especially recent memory) and a disordered sense of time. The patient has islets of preserved memory but may not be able to put these memories into the correct time sequence. Thus he may recall a remote event but describe it as though it occurred recently. Gaps in memory may be filled by making details up (confabulation).

Peripheral neuropathy is a feature. Patients are anxious, tachycardic, and have sweating with tremor and sometimes pyrexia. Clouding of consciousness suggests an acute confusional state.

Tutorial

Causes of Korsakoff's syndrome:
- Alcohol.
- Thiamine deficiency.
- Subarachnoid haemorrhage.
- Meningovascular syphilis.
- Intracranial tumour.

Other neuropsychiatric complications of alcoholism:
- Wernicke's encephalopathy.
- Dementia (unlike other forms of dementia, progression is not inevitable and cognition may improve on abstinence).

Answer 9

B Hopelessness.

There are no symptoms that are pathognomonic of schizophrenia, but in practice the Schneiderian first rank symptoms (e.g. thought blocking) enable classification. Delusions of grandeur are not something that depressed individuals are familiar with! Delusions of passivity include delusions of control, such as one's belief that one's will is being taken over by some alien force. Anxiety and hopelessness are suggestive of a depressive illness.

Question 10 The following is characteristic of an obsessional neurosis:

A Hyperventilation attacks.
B Intrusive thoughts attributed by the patient to some external agency.
C Fuges.
D Rumination.
E Successful resistance to repeated antisocial impulses.

Question 11 Paranoid delusions are not a recognized feature of:

A Senile dementia.
B Schizophrenia.
C Obsessional states.
D Depressive psychosis.
E Amphetamine.

Question 12 Mental retardation is an expected finding in:

A Glycogen storage disease.
B Alcaptonuria.
C Lactose intolerance.
D Maple syrup urine disease.
E Cystinuria.

Question 13 The following would be an unusual finding in obsessional neurosis:

A Patients have good insight.
B Patients often give way to their aggressive impulses.
C Depression is to be expected.
D Inconclusive rumination is characteristic.
E Frustration.

Answer 10

D Rumination.

Obsessional neurosis (obsessive compulsive disorder):
- The incidence is equal for men and women.
- It is a rare disorder (0.1–2.0/1000).
- The course is characterized by remissions and exacerbations and treatment is usually difficult. Behavioural techniques (response prevention) can be of use.

Ruminations are based on the patient endlessly and pointlessly reviewing even the simplest everyday event.

Hyperventilation occurs in anxiety neurosis. Thought insertion occurs in schizophrenia. Impulses are not usually antisocial.

Answer 11

C Obsessional states.

Paranoid delusions occur in schizophrenia, depressive psychosis as opposed to depressive neurosis, substance abuse, and senile dementia. Paranoid delusions are not a feature of neurosis.

Answer 12

D Maple syrup urine disease.

Specific aetiological factors for mental retardation include:
- Genetic or chromosomal (maple syrup disease, phenylketonuria, Down's syndrome).
- Abnormalities in prenatal environment (rubella during pregnancy, maternal alcoholism, rhesus incompatibility).
- Trauma during birth or early infancy (mechanical injury during delivery, hypoxia, status epilepticus).

Intellect is preserved in alcaptonuria, glycogen storage disease, lactose intolerance, and cystinuria.

Answer 13

B Patients often give way to their aggressive impulses.

In obsessional neurosis:
- Patients have good insight.
- Depression is to be expected.
- Inconclusive rumination is characteristic.

This is a frequent topic for MRCP 1! In obsessional neurosis, impulses are not aggressive.

Question 14 A 50-year-old male becomes progressively more uncommunicative and withdrawn. A diagnosis of dementia rather than depression is supported by:

A Sexual impotence.
B Faecal incontinence.
C Mutism.
D Marked impairment of concentration.
E Early morning wakening.

Question 15 The following would make the diagnosis of early schizophrenia unlikely:

A Depersonalization.
B Feeling of being under an occult force.
C Moving residence.
D Persistent headache.
E Blunting of emotional response.

Question 16 Recognized causes of severe memory loss for recent events include the following with the exception of:

A Hysteria (dissociated type).
B HIV infection.
C Cardiac surgery.
D Head injury.
E Depressive psychosis.

Question 17 Adverse effects of cannabis do not include:

A Panic attacks.
B Reduced spermatogenesis.
C Visual hallucinations.
D Flashbacks.
E Physical dependence.

Question 18 The following is not associated with alcoholism:

A Auditory hallucinations in a clear consciousness.
B Deliberate self harm.
C Morbid jealousy.
D Dysphoria.
E Domestic harmony.

Answer 14

B Faecal incontinence.

Faecal incontinence and antisocial behaviour occur in dementia. Impotence is a feature of depression. Depressed patients are usually constipated with impaired concentration, and in severe cases become mute.

Answer 15

E Blunting of emotional response.

Depersonalization is a sense that one is 'unreal'. It is not uncommon in the general population, especially at times of stress. It also occurs in early schizophrenia, anxiety, and depression. Persistent headache suggests an organic disorder.

Tutorial

Schizophrenia:

- The lifetime risk is 1% (higher in western Ireland, northern Sweden, and Yugoslavia).
- The onset is earlier in men (peak 3rd decade) than women (peak 4th decade).
- Patients are more likely to be born in winter months.
- The concordance in monozygote twins is 50%.
- The risk to a child born to a schizophrenic is 12%.

Answer 16

E Depressive psychosis.

Cardiac surgery is a rare cause of recent memory loss.

Recent memory is not impaired in psychotic illness, although delusions may alter interpretation.

Answer 17

E Physical dependence.

Panic attacks may occur during intoxication. The effects of the drug are more commonly feelings of euphoria, relaxation, and subjective feelings of well-being. Perceptual disturbances may occur and, rarely, visual hallucinations.

Physiological effects of cannabis include reduced body temperature, increased appetite, and reduced sperm count. Transient flashback phenomena may occur, in which the individual may experience the effects of intoxication well beyond the time the drug was taken. Psychological dependence is well documented.

Answer 18

E Domestic harmony.

Alcoholism is associated with an increased prevalence of functional psychiatric disorders. Irritability and dysphoria are common and may be mistaken for depressive illness. There is an increased incidence of self harm. Ten to fifteen percent of completed suicides have a history of alcoholism.

Alcohol is a common concomitant of marital violence (50% of battered wives reporting their husband as a heavy drinker). Morbid jealousy is another association, in which the patient has a delusional belief that his spouse is being unfaithful to him. A variety of sexual problems occur including impotence and exhibitionism due to the disinhibitant effects of alcohol.

Alcoholic hallucinosis is a rare complication in which the patient has auditory hallucinations in clear consciousness. They usually resolve after a few days of abstinence.

Question 19 Suicide risk is not increased in:

A History of alcohol abuse.
B Epilepsy.
C History of obsessional neurosis.
D Old age.
E Being socially isolated.

Question 20 The following statement is not true of puerperal (post-natal) psychosis:

A 1/200 mothers is affected.
B The onset of symptoms is usually within 2 days of delivery.
C Is more common in single parent mothers.
D Appropriate treatment may include ECT.
E There is an increased risk for mothers who have suffered from puerperal depression in previous pregnancies.

Answer 19

C History of obsessional neurosis.

Suicide is increased in:

- Men.
- Social isolation.
- Recent divorce or bereavement.
- Depression.
- Alcoholism.
- Chronic illness (renal dialysis >400-fold risk, epilepsy fivefold risk).

The suicide rate is actually low in patients with obsessional neurosis.

Answer 20

B The onset of symptoms is usually within 2 days of delivery.

Puerperal psychosis is typically of acute onset, often following two or more sleepless nights. Psychotic manifestations do not become apparent immediately and may take up to 2 weeks to develop. Symptoms very seldom start within the first 2 days of delivery.

Treatment is based on keeping mother and baby together if possible. ECT is safer than oral medication if the mother is breastfeeding. There is often a family history or a past personal history of psychosis. Having had one episode of puerperal psychosis increases the future risk from 1/200 to 1/7.

11 Renal medicine

Question 1 A 60-year-old male presents with a 1-month history of loin pain. On examination blood +++ on a urine dipstick and an abdominal mass. The following would make a diagnosis of hypernephroma unlikely:

A He has large lesions on his chest X-ray.
B He has a left-sided varicocoele.
C He has a high ESR.
D He has a raised serum aldosterone.
E He is pyrexial.

Question 2 The following is true for acute tubular necrosis:

A Rarely presents with anuria of acute onset.
B Is unlikely to complicate major trauma.
C The urinary sodium concentration is characteristically <50 mmol/l.
D Selective mild proteinuria is a feature.
E The urine plasma osmolality ratio is <1:1.

Question 3 The following are recognized causes of metabolic acidosis with a high anion gap with the exception of:

A Ureterosigmoidostomy.
B Diabetic ketoacidosis.
C Salicylate intoxication.
D Vitamin D intoxication.
E Methanol administration.

Answer 1

D He has a raised serum aldosterone.

Hypernephroma is more common in males, with a male to female ratio of 2:1. The tumour may spread locally to involve the renal veins and as the left testicular vein drains directly into the renal vein, the carcinoma may rarely be complicated by a left-sided varicocoele. A high ESR is characteristic and several hormones may be secreted, namely renin (causing hypokalaemia and hypertension), PTHrP (causing humoral hypercalcaemia of malignancy), ADH (SIADH), and erythropoetin causing polcythaemia. Pyrogens are also secreted resulting in a pyrexia of unknown origin.

Tutorial

Clinical features of hypernephroma consist of a triad of loin pain, haematuria, and an abdominal mass. Haematogenous spread occurs to bone, liver, and lung (cannon ball lesions on CXR). Peak age of presentation is 40–60 years with a 5-year survival of 30–50%.

Histology
Solid and clear cell types are often found in the same tumour. Most patients with cancer have a fever at some time during the course of their illness. This fever may be due to concomitant infection, localized obstruction by the tumour, surgery, and post-operative complications, or by the neoplasm itself.

Neoplasms most frequently associated with PUO:
- Hodgkin's disease.
- Non-Hodgkin's lymphoma.
- Leukaemia.
- Hepatoma.
- Hypernephroma.

Less frequent: solid tumours such as carcinoma of the:
- Stomach.
- Pancreas.
- Colon.
- Breast.
- Hepatic metastases.

Other malignant tumours of the kidney:
- Nephroblastoma.
- Transitional cell carcinoma of the renal pelvis.
- Squamous cell carcinoma of the renal pelvis (rare).
- Sarcoma (rare).

Answer 2

E The urine plasma osmolality ratio is <1:1.

Acute tubular necrosis is characterized by acute oliguric, potentially reversible, renal failure. It may complicate major trauma (crush syndrome in World War II). Other causes include ischaemia, cardiogenic and septic shock, tubular toxins (Bence Jones' proteins, contrast, and myoglobin), drugs such as gentamicin, and acute pancreatitis.

Investigations show:
- Urine osmolality is low <350 mmol/kg
- Urine plasma to creatinine ratio <20:1.
- Urine sodium >50 mmol/l.
- Urine to plasma osmolality ratio <1:1.

Tutorial

The oliguria develops over 1–5 days and lasts on average 11 days. There is a mild unselective proteinuria and urine microscopy shows red cell and granular casts. In cases of extensive tissue damage, life-threatening hyperkalaemia may occur. Maximal recovery of renal function is in the range of 80%, which usually occurs in the first year.

Pathological features include swelling and pallor of the kidneys, with tubular epithelial necrosis. Calcium oxalate crystals may be found in the lumen.

If the patient has received diuretic therapy the interpretation of the above results is invalidated.

Answer 3

A Ureterosigmoidostomy.

Tutorial

Drug causes of metabolic acidosis with high anion gap include:
- Salicylates.
- Methanol.
- Ethylene glycol.
- Paraldehyde.

Causes of metabolic acidosis with a normal anion gap include:
- Loss of HCO_3: diarrhoea, ureterosigmoidostomy, pancreatic fistula.
- Renal tubular acidosis: proximal and distal types.
- Rapid IV hydration.
- Acetozolamide treatment.
- Excess cationic amino acids in feeds.

Metabolic acidosis with a high anion gap may occur in uraemia secondary to renal disease where there is reduced filtration of PO_4 and impaired production of NH_3 leading to failed excretion of H^+ and acidosis. This may also be seen in vitamin D intoxication.

In ketoacidosis the high anion gap is due to accumulation of organic acids. It may complicate IDDM (diabetic ketoacidosis), ethanol intoxication, and starvation.

Lactic acidosis should be suspected in patients where there is a high anion gap acidosis with no evidence of uraemia or DKA. Lactic acidosis type A occurs when production of lactate is increased and peripheral breakdown reduced, e.g. in shock, strenuous exercise, and severe hypoxia. Patients with liver and renal disease are more prone to lactic acidosis of this type due to impaired metabolism and excretion.

Lactic acidosis type B can also produce this picture and is a result of drugs and toxins (e.g. phenformin, less frequently metformin, alcohol, and paracetamol intoxication), leukaemia, and TPN with fructose or sorbitol.

Question 4 The following is not true for Goodpasture's syndrome:

A The anti-GBM antibody is of the IgG type.
B High antibody titres are associated with rapid onset of end-stage renal failure.
C 90% of patients have HLA DR2.
D Lung haemorrhage is more common in smokers.
E Lung haemorrhage responds well to plasmapheresis.

Question 5 The following is not true for minimal change glomerulonephritis:

A Is more common in children under 5 years of age.
B Is the commonest cause of nephrotic syndrome.
C May present with hypertension.
D Corticosteroids are the treatment of choice.
E Affected individuals have a high incidence of atopy.

Question 6 The following is not a recognized cause of aminoaciduria:

A Phenylketonuria.
B Hartnup disease.
C Chronic liver disease.
D Haemachromatosis.
E Galactosaemia.

Answer 4

B High antibody titres are associated with rapid onset of end-stage renal failure.

In Goodpasture's syndrome the anti-GBM antibody is of the IgG type and is directed at shared antigens on the glomerular basement membranes and alveolar capillary basement membranes. The resultant syndrome is one of recurrent haemoptysis and a severe proliferative glomerulonephritis. Clinical progression is rapid, many patients die within the first 6 months; high antibody titres are not related to the rate of demise. Respiratory symptoms precede renal failure and usually manifest as an upper respiratory tract infection associated with SOB and haemoptysis due to intrapulmonary haemorrhage.

Ninety percent of patients have HLA DR2 although it is the presence of the HLA B7 that is associated with severe disease. Pulmonary haemorrhage occurs in 60% of patients and is much more common amongst smokers. Lung haemorrhage responds to repeated plasmapheresis which removes the antibody, and the severity of the disease can be modified by immunosuppressants.

The influenza A2 virus has an association via a probable shared antigen, with both basement membranes leading to a type II cytotoxic hypersensitivity reaction. In this condition the anaemia is out of proportion with the degree of renal impairment.

Answer 5

C May present with hypertension.

Minimal change glomerulonephritis is more common in the 2–4 year age group, accounting for 80% of cases of nephrotic syndrome in this group. Affected individuals have a higher incidence of atopy.

In Africa and other endemic areas malaria is the most common cause of nephrotic states in this age group. Minimal change accounts for 20% of cases of nephrotic syndrome in adults. Hypertension is not a feature and the condition does not progress to chronic renal failure. Proteinuria is selective and complement levels are normal.

The condition is associated with Hodgkin's lymphoma and also amyloidosis. The aetiology is thought to be a reaction to lymphokines produced as a hypersensitivity response to toxins, insect stings, pollens, and foodstuffs. Light microscopy is normal and electron microscopy reveals fusion of the podocytes (foot processes).

Corticosteroids are the treatment of choice allowing for remission in 90% of cases, although patients who relapse frequently (25%) may respond to cyclophosphamide, which offers long periods of remission.

Answer 6

D Haemachromatosis.

Conditions associated with aminoaciduria are:

- Overflow due to plasma levels above the renal threshold.
- Liver failure.
- Phenylketonuria.
- Histidinaemia.
- Maple syrup urine.
- Fanconi syndrome.
- Lowe's syndrome (mental retardation, congenital cataracts, generalized aminoaciduria, hypotonia).
- Methionine malabsorption syndrome (impaired absorption and excretion of methionine), resulting in vomiting, diarrhoea, mental retardation, and oat house smell).
- Blue diaper syndrome (specific for trytophan which is oxidized on the nappy giving a blue colour).

Tutorial

Healthy individuals lose trace amounts of alanine, glycine, serine, histidine, and glutamine in urine. Hartnup's disease (autosomal recessive, selective) is characterized by defective absorption at the jejunum and the proximal tubule. There is, as a result, malabsorption of neutral amino acids, the most important of which is tryptophan, producing nicotinamide deficiency and in some cases pellagra.

Cystinuria is caused by a similar mechanism (inheritance is complete or incomplete AR, selective). It results in the formation of renal stones. Treatment consists of drinking at least 3 litres of fluid daily, and penicillamine is reserved for those who do not respond to this measure.

Fanconi syndrome is a well recognized cause of defective tubular absorption of most amino acids and may be caused by galactosaemia, Wilson's disease, cystinosis, myeloma, lead poisoning, and post-renal transplantation.

Question 7 The following is not true for adult polycystic kidney disease:

A Is inherited as an autosomal dominant disorder.
B May be complicated by polycythaemia.
C Hepatic cysts are seen in 10% of patients.
D May be complicated by renal carcinoma.
E Urinary tract infections are difficult to treat.

Question 8 The presence of the following in the urinary sediment indicate significant renal pathology with the exception of:

A Red cell casts.
B Hyaline casts.
C Epithelial cell casts.
D White cell casts.
E Large wide cell casts.

Question 9 The following is not true for membranous glomerulonephritis:

A When idiopathic carries a worse prognosis on males.
B May complicate successful renal transplant for Alport's syndrome.
C Is associated with atopy.
D Spontaneous remission is more common in women.
E Is associated with HLA DR3.

Question 10 The following are recognized complications of haemodialysis with the exception of:

A Amyloidosis.
B Myoclonic spasms.
C Bacterial endocarditis.
D High output cardiac failure.
E Hypotriglyceridaemia.

Answer 7

C Hepatic cysts are seen in 10% of patients.

Adult polycystic disease is autosomal dominant. Polycythaemia is secondary to increased erythropoetin production. Thirty percent of patients have co-existing hepatic cysts which rarely cause liver dysfunction. Occasionally, carcinoma may develop within the cysts and diagnosis in this situation is very difficult. Urinary tract infections are often recurrent and particularly difficult to treat. There is a well-known association with berry aneurysms and intracranial haemorrhage.

Hypertension should be treated vigorously as it accelerates loss of renal function. On intravenous pyelogram, grossly enlarged kidneys with spidery calyces are virtually pathognomonic of polycystic kidney disease.

Medullary cystic disease developing in early childhood is autosomal recessive.

Answer 8

B Hyaline casts.

Casts are cylindrical structures formed by the moulding of cells or proteins in the distal tubular lumen. Red cell casts always indicate renal disease and occur in glomerulonephritis. Coarse granular casts occur with pathological proteinuria and may be numerous in acute tubular necrosis. White cell casts commonly occur in pyelonephritis.

Epithelial cells are a normal finding in the urinary sediment although the development of casts usually signifies inflammation. They may also occur in oliguric renal failure. Wide cell casts are formed in the larger ducts and imply significant renal impairment.

Hyaline casts and fine granular casts represent precipitated protein and may be seen in healthy individuals, especially after exercise and sometimes following a febrile illness.

Answer 9

C Is associated with atopy.

There are many associations with membranous glomerulonephritis but idiopathic cases are commoner and carry a worse prognosis in males. Membranous GN can affect the disease-free transplanted kidneys of patients who have had transplant for Alport's syndrome, although the latter does not recur. There is a strong association with HLA DR3.

Atopy is more common in patients with minimal change. Spontaneous remission occurs in 30% of adults, and is more common in women.

Associated conditions include SLE, malignancy (mainly bowel and bronchus), *Plasmodium malariae*, penicillamine, gold, and mercury. It is an insidious disorder presenting with proteinuria or frank nephrotic syndrome.

- Light microscopy – thickening of the basement membrane.
- Electron microscopy – subepithelial deposits (IgG and C3).

Answer 10

E Hypotriglyceridaemia.

Haemodialysis with cuprophane allows accumulation of beta-2-microglobulin and the development of dialysis related amyloid. This may be complicated by entrapment neuropathy, e.g. carpal tunnel syndrome.

Aluminium toxicity was once common when aluminium containing phosphate binders were used in dialysis. Nowadays toxicity is seen in areas where aluminium salts are added to local water as flocculating agents. Toxicity is associated with:

- Hypochromic microcytic anaemia (due to interference with haem biosynthesis).
- Vitamin D resistance, osteomalacia, and multiple fractures.
- Dialysis dementia, dysarthria, ataxia, myoclonus, and seizures.

Bacterial endocarditis can occur as a result of central line infection. Fistulas may cause high output cardiac failure. Multiple renal cysts can complicate up to 40% of patients who have been dialysed for many years. Neoplasms occur in up to 30% of patients with such cysts, 10% of these are malignant.

Patients on HD retain certain substances that are normally metabolized by the kidney, resulting in elevated levels of gastrin and hence an increased incidence of PUD, and also increased PTH which may cause itching. The latter symptom may be worsened acutely during dialysis.

Tutorial

Acute and subacute complications of haemodialysis:

- Hyper- or hypotension (may be complicated by hypertensive encephalopathy).
- Angina, arrhythmia.
- Fluid overload and heart failure.
- Leucopenia (transient, may be severe).
- Thrombocytopenia (mild but progressive).
- Haemorrhage.
- Haemolysis.
- Anaphylaxis.
- Hypercalcaemia.
- Hypermagnesaemia.
- Hyper- or hypokalaemia.
- Hyper- or hyponatraemia.
- Air embolism.
- Priapism.

Chronic complications of haemodialysis:

- Anaemia.
- Hypertension.
- Ischaemic heart disease.
- Peripheral neuropathy.
- Carpal tunnel syndrome.
- Thiamine deficiency.
- Hyperparathyroidism.
- Osteomalacia.
- Raised triglycerides with type IV hyperlipidaemia.
- Increased gastrin, growth hormone, glucagons, and melanocyte stimulating hormone.
- Infertility.

Question 11 Renal damage is a recognized complication of infection with the following with the exception of:

A *Plasmodium falciparum*.
B *Schistosoma mansoni*.
C *Plasmodium malariae*.
D *Leptospira icterhaemorrhagica*.
E *Mycobacterium leprae*.

Question 12 An increase in the ratio of plasma urea to creatinine occurs in:

A Psychogenic polydipsia.
B Low protein diet.
C Corticosteroid therapy.
D Liver failure.
E SIADH production.

Question 13 Glomerulonephritis and low serum complement do not occur in:

A Goodpasture's syndrome.
B SLE.
C Bacterial endocarditis.
D Mesangiocapillary glomerulonephritis.
E Penicillamine therapy.

Answer 11

B *Schistosoma mansoni.*

Renal damage is associated with all of the infective agents listed with the exception of *S. mansoni.*

Plasmodium malariae is a common cause of membranous glomerulonephritis in the tropics. *P. falciparum* is associated with high levels of parasitaemia, and the infected RBCs develop knob-like projections, which facilitate adhesion to the endothelium of blood vessels and predispose to occlusion. This can result in severe organ damage especially renal, brain, and GI tract.

Schistosoma haematobium predominantly affects the urinary system. It commonly produces chronic inflammation of the bladder, ureters, and urethra causing dysuria, frequency, and haematuria. Chronic infection produces an obstructive uropathy, chronic pyelonephritis, renal failure, and contraction of the bladder. There is an association with bladder carcinoma.

Leptospira icterhaemorrhagica causes Weil's disease and is acquired from leptospires excreted in animal urine. The disease consists of jaundice, renal impairment, and haemorrhage, although fever, conjunctivitis, meningitis, cough with sputum, and haematuria may occur. In 85% of patients the illness is self-limiting without jaundice.

Lepromatous leprosy can affect virtually any organ. In the kidneys this may manifest as a glomerulonephritis or calcification.

Answer 12

C Corticosteroid therapy.

Plasma creatinine is dependent on two main factors, both of which are fairly constant on a day-to-day basis. These are GFR and skeletal muscle mass. Plasma urea is variable and production is increased in catabolic states, e.g. infection, steroids, and tissue injury. In GI haemorrhage, there is ingestion of large amounts of nitrogen from the breakdown of blood. Similar situations arise from a high protein diet and uretocolic anastomosis. In SIADH there is haemodilution and hence plasma urea falls. In liver disease there is impaired production of urea. In dehydration, e.g. pyloric stenosis and diarrhoea, urea excretion falls due to increased tubular reabsorption.

Answer 13

A Goodpasture's syndrome.

Tutorial

Effects of penicillamine on the kidneys:

- An immune complex-mediated membranous glomerulonephritis.
- SLE-like syndrome with renal involvement.
- Goodpasture's syndrome.
- Nephrotic syndrome.
- Haematuria.

Glomerulonephritis and low serum complement can be caused by renal involvement in SLE, and is 10-fold more common in females. It can cause all types of glomerulonephritis and is associated with reduced C3 in most cases, with the exception of minimal change where complement is normal. In bacterial endocarditis, total serum complement and C3 is reduced as a result of immune complex disease.

Mesangiocapillary glomerulonephritis may be associated with the presence of C3 nephritic factor, which is an IgG autoantibody that stabilizes C3 convertase in the complement cascade, allowing continuous degradation of C3.

Serum complement levels are generally normal in Goodpasture's syndrome.

Question 14 The following is true for myoglobinuria:

A May complicate hyperkalaemia.
B Urine dipstick is positive for blood and red cells.
C Senile immobility is a recognized cause.
D Frusemide diuresis is a recognized treatment.
E Serum aldolase is characteristically raised.

Question 15 The following is true for hepatorenal syndrome:

A Most frequently complicates gall bladder surgery.
B Serum sodium is >120 mmol/l.
C Renal transplant is the treatment of choice.
D Oliguria is characteristic.
E Plasma expanders may improve renal function in volume depleted patients.

Question 16 A male aged 40 years is found to be uraemic. The following facts might give a useful lead to the aetiology with the exception of:

A He had severe and recurrent tonsillitis in childhood.
B He works in an iron foundry.
C Three of his children had haemolytic disease of the newborn.
D He has taken tablets regularly for fibrositis.
E He suffers from migraine.

Question 17 The following is not true for Fanconi syndrome:

A Is associated with glycosuria.
B May be complicated by mental retardation.
C Can cause hypophosphataemic rickets.
D Can be treated by replacement therapy.
E May complicate lead toxicity.

Answer 14

E Serum aldolase is characteristically raised.

Myoglobinuria is often asymptomatic. Serum aldolase and CK are high. Hypokalaemia can predispose to myoglobinuria. Acute renal failure complicates myoglobinuria, and may be associated with markedly raised potassium and phosphate if there is massive tissue breakdown. Frusemide should be avoided as it may acidify the urine and precipitate myoglobin.

Mannitol diuresis is the treatment of choice, along with alkalinization of the urine with intravenous bicarbonate. Dialysis may be necessary. Urine should be checked for myoglobin within the first 48 hours and is positive for blood in the absence of RBC.

Causes of myoglobinuria:

- Crush injury.
- Exercise.
- Trauma associated with muscle injury or necrosis.
- Burns.
- Electric shock.
- Coma.
- Sepsis.
- Seizures.
- Hypokalaemia.

Answer 15

D Oliguria is characteristic.

Hepatorenal syndrome typically follows surgery to the lower bile duct to relieve long standing jaundice. It may also complicate end-stage alcoholic cirrhosis. The underlying mechanism is thought to be changes in renal blood flow resulting in cortical hypoperfusion. It is characterized by oliguria, serum sodium of <120 mmol/l, and urinary sodium of <10 mmol/l. The kidneys are histologically normal and will function if transplanted into a recipient with a functioning liver.

Liver transplant is the treatment of choice. Although blood volume is reduced, plasma expanders rarely improve renal function. The condition can be prevented by mannitol diuresis before and during surgery.

Answer 16

B He works in an iron foundry.

This male may have analgesic nephropathy as a result of taking NSAIDs for fibrositis and migraine. Ergometrine used for migraine may cause retroperitoneal fibrosis, and hence obstructive uropathy.

Haemolytic disease of the newborn is caused by the passage of IgG from the maternal circulation via the placenta to the foetus, where it causes destruction of foetal red blood cells. It is caused by incompatibilities in the rhesus blood group system.

Answer 17

B May be complicated by mental retardation.

Fanconi's syndrome is a disorder characterized by multiple proximal tubule defects.

Tutorial

Proximal tubule defects include:
- Glycosuria.
- Aminoaciduria.
- Phosphaturia, resulting in hypophosphataemic rickets.
- RTA due to excretion of HCO_3 producing a hyperchloraemic acidosis.
- Hypouricaemia.
- Hypokalaemia causing weakness.
- Polyuria leading to dehydration.
- Excretion of immunoglobulins.

Juvenile form (cystinosis): presentation at 6–9 months with:
- Vomiting.
- Thirst.
- Failure to thrive.
- Dehydration and acidosis.
- Associated with vitamin D resistant rickets.
- Renal failure occurs before age 10 years.
- Treatment is with HCO_3, K^+, PO_4, and ergocalciferol.
- Cystamine may halt progression.

Adult form (idiopathic):
This is similar to the juvenile form, but back pain caused by osteomalacia is a major feature. Treatment is with large doses of vitamin D with regular calcium monitoring.

Secondary Fanconi's syndrome may occur following:
- Renal transplantation.
- Lead poisoning.
- Wilson's disease.
- Myeloma.
- Out-of-date tetracyclines.
- Vitamin D deficiency.
- Hypokalaemia.
- Galactosaemia.
- Fructose intolerance.

Question 18 The following is not true for nephrotic syndrome:

A Renal vein thrombosis is a recognized complication.
B May be complicated by acute tubular necrosis.
C Hypercholesterolaemia is characteristic.
D Renal tuberculosis is a recognized cause.
E Patients are more prone to septicaemia.

Question 19 The following are true for xanthogranulomatous pyelonephritis with the exception of:

A Is caused by proteus infection.
B May present with fever and weight loss.
C Usually affects both kidneys.
D CT scanning reveals intrarenal abscesses.
E Nephrectomy is the treatment of choice.

Question 20 The following is not true for contrast nephropathy:

A Is more common in diabetic patients.
B Is more likely to occur when the blood pressure is not controlled.
C Can be prevented by intravenous dopamine infusion.
D Is more likely in patients with salt and water depletion.
E May also occur with the use of nonionic contrast.

Answer 18

D Renal tuberculosis is a recognized cause.

Nephrotic syndrome consists of a triad of heavy proteinuria (3–5 g/24 hrs), hypoalbuminaemia (usually <20 g/l), and oedema. Hypercholesterolaemia frequently occurs but is not invariably present. Patients are more prone to septicaemia as a result of loss of globulins, and bronchopneumonia is a common cause of death.

There is an increased risk of thromboembolic complications (5–50%), and renal vein thrombosis is recognized as a complication rather than a cause of nephrotic syndrome. Embolic disease most frequently complicates nephrotic syndrome caused by membranous GN.

A low blood volume and hypotension may result in hypoperfusion of the kidneys resulting in acute tubular necrosis.

Renal TB is associated with proteinuria but this is not sufficient to produce the nephrotic state.

Tutorial

Causes of nephrotic syndrome:

- All types of glomerulonephritis.
- Minimal change 50% in childhood, 20% in adults.
- Membranous, also caused by SLE, malaria, penicillamine, malignancy, hepatitis B.
- Diabetic glomerulosclerosis.
- Drugs:
  - Penicillamine.
  - Troxidone.
- Gold, mercury, cadmium (produce membranous GN).
- Allergies:
  - Poison ivy.
  - Bee sting.
- Haematological malignancies.
- Myeloma.
- Hodgkin's disease.
- Amyloidosis.
- Infections:
  - Staphylococcal septicaemia.
  - Syphilis.
  - Bacterial endocarditis.
  - CMV.
  - Leprosy.
  - Smallpox vaccination.
- Renal artery stenosis.
- Constrictive pericarditis.

Several renal disorders are associated with proteinuria not severe enough to produce nephrotic syndrome. These are:

- Chronic tubulointerstitial nephritis.
- Renal TB.
- Polycystic kidneys.
- Renal papillary necrosis.
- Reflux nephropathy and pyelonephritis.
- Obstructive cardiac failure.
- Postural proteinuria.

Causes of renal vein thrombosis:

- Nephrotic syndrome.
- Renal amyloidosis.
- Hypernephroma.
- Dehydration.
- Trauma including cannulation.

Answer 19

C Usually affects both kidneys.

Xanthogranulomatous pyelonephritis is a rare condition caused by proteus infection. Symptoms include:

- Loin pain.
- Fever.
- Weight loss.

It is usually unilateral and may be complicated by the development of a stag horn calculus. Examination may reveal a tender enlarged kidney. CT scan shows multiple lucent areas in the kidney, which are intrarenal abscesses.

Antibiotics are seldom effective in eradication of infection, and nephrectomy is the treatment of choice.

Answer 20

C Can be prevented by intravenous dopamine infusion.

Contrast nephropathy is more common in diabetic patients and those with generalized atheromatous disease. It can be prevented to some extent by ensuring adequate hydration and blood pressure control.

Dopamine infusions have not been shown to reduce the incidence in high risk patients.

12 Respiratory Medicine

A 60-year-old builder presents with a 12-month history of progressive dyspnoea. He has seen his GP on many occasions during this time and has been treated with inhalers, several courses of antibiotics, and high doses of steroids. He is a lifelong smoker, smoking 20–30 cigarettes a day. On examination he is thin, plethoric, and has finger clubbing. Examination of his respiratory system reveals reduced expansion of both lung fields, resonant percussion, and bilateral inspiratory crepitations at both lung bases. A chest X-ray shows hyperinflation of the lung fields with evidence of pleural plaques and calcification. There is also a small left-sided pleural effusion. Results: FEV1 1.9 l; FEVC 2.4 l; FEV1/FVC 78%.

Question 1 The most likely cause of his condition is:

A Carcinoma of the bronchus.
B Asbestosis.
C Cryptogenic fibrosing alveolitis.
D Sarcoidosis.
E Obstructive airways disease.

A 65-year-old female with a long history of atrial fibrillation presents with a 5-month history of progressive lethargy and shortness of breath. She describes symptoms of depression and impaired concentration. She has also noticed that her skin is very dry. On examination she has multiple skin excoriations of her forehead, which she attributes to sunbathing recently. She also has bilateral widespread fine respiratory crackles throughout her lung fields.

Question 2 The most likely cause of her symptoms is:

A Primary hypothyroidism.
B Dementia.
C Depression.
D Long-term treatment with amiodarone.
E Connective tissue disease.

A 40-year-old female, nonsmoker, presents to Accident & Emergency with severe breathlessness. Arterial blood gases confirm a PaO_2 of 60 mmHg (8.0 kPa). Lung function tests confirm normal lung volumes but a reduced TLCO at 50% of predicted.

Question 3 The least likely diagnosis is:

A Pneumonectomy.
B Anaemia.
C Left ventricular failure.
D Goodpasture's syndrome.
E Pulmonary AV malformation.

Answer 1

B Asbestosis.

The lung pathology on exposure to asbestos consists of fibrosis and hence a restrictive defect is to be expected. As with other causes of interstitial lung diseases, gas transfer is reduced.The investigation of choice is high resolution CT scan.

The pleura and peritoneum are identical structures and peritoneal mesothelioma is a recognized complication. Carcinoma of the bladder is associated with chronic inflammation of the bladder, exposure to alanine dyes, and is more common in smokers. Fibrosis is more prominent in the subpleural regions of the lower lobes.

Tutorial

Asbestosis can be defined as diffuse pulmonary parenchymal interstitial fibrosis secondary to the inhalation of asbestos fibres. It results from heavy exposure and because the fibres remain impacted, the disease often occurs long after exposure has ceased (5–20 years).

There are three types of asbestos fibre:

- Chrysolite (white asbestos): 90%. Fibres are 2 cm long but only a few micrometres thick. They are fibrogenic, but far less than crocidolite fibres.
- Crocidolite (blue asbestos): 6%. Straight fibres 50 µm long and 1–2 µm thick which are particularly resistant to chemical, macrophage, and neutrophil enzyme destruction. Fibres are easily inhaled and impacted in the bronchioli. By far the most important type in the development of asbestosis and mesothelioma.
- Amosite: 4%. Not important in pathogenesis.

Symptoms are those of progressive dyspnoea. There is a synergistic relationship with smoking, with a fivefold increase in adenocarcinoma of the bronchus.

Pulmonary function tests show:

- Restrictive defect with preservation of ventilatory function.
- Reduced vital capacity.
- Reduced residual volume.
- Reduced transfer factor.
- Hypoxemia on exercise (PCO_2 is usually normal or low).

Asbestosis may be complicated by:

- Shortness of breath.
- Cough (dry or productive of mucopurulent sputum).
- Clubbing (30–40%)*.
- Lung fibrosis with pleural plaques.
- Honeycomb lung.
- Mesothelioma.
- Adenocarcinoma.
- Pleural effusion (usually benign).

*Clubbing in asbestosis occurs early in the disease process and predicts a greater likelihood of progression of disease to pulmonary fibrosis. It is associated with a higher mortality rate but is not associated with heavy exposure.

Answer 2

D Long-term treatment with amiodarone.

Tutorial

Drugs that may produce pulmonary shadowing with an eosinophilia:

- Aspirin.
- Nitrofurantoin.
- Methotrexate.
- Phenylbutazone.
- Rifampicin.

Busulphan and cyclophosphamide may also produce a dilated cardiomyopathy. Phenylbutazone may cause bilateral hilar lymphadenopathy which is difficult to differentiate from sarcoidosis.

The following drugs can all produce diffuse lung disease closely resembling cryptogenic fibrosing alveolitis:

- Amiodarone.
- Nitrofurantoin.
- Cyclophosphamide.
- Chlorambucil.
- Procarbazine.
- Sulphasalazine.
- Busulphan.
- Bleomycin.
- Methotrexate.
- Paraquat (found in weed killer) produces an acute and progressive rapidly fatal lung fibrosis.

Cryptogenic fibrosing alveolitis itself is a rare disorder of unknown aetiology which usually occurs after the fourth decade and is associated with generalized lung fibrosis.

Answer 3

D Goodpasture's syndrome.

A reduced transfer factor is found in:
- Pneumonectomy.
- Anaemia.
- Left ventricular failure.

Gas transfer is normal in asthmatics.

Pulmonary AV malformations cause right to left shunts thus reducing TLCO values and provoking hypoxaemia. Polycythaemia and pulmonary haemorrhage syndromes usually cause elevation of TLCO.

Tutorial

Transfer factor is a measure of transfer of carbon monoxide across the lung, hence the use of TLCO. It is measured by inhaling 0.3% of CO and measuring the expired gas after 10 seconds. Measurement of alveolar volume (VA) by helium dilution is done at the same time.

TLCO depends on:
- Alveolar volume.
- Thickness of the alveolar capillary membrane.
- VQ imbalance and the presence of blood or lack of it in the capillaries and bronchial tree.

Reduced TLCO is seen in:
- Pneumonectomy.
- Interstitial lung disease (due to destruction of gas exchange surface), e.g. cryptogenic fibrosing alveolitis.
- Sarcoidosis.
- Asbestosis.
- Multiple pulmonary emboli.
- Emphysema.
- Anaemia.
- LVF.
- Right-to-left shunt (reduced pulmonary blood flow, pulmonary HT, and VQ mismatch).

Increased TLCO is seen in:
- Men.
- Athletes.
- During childhood.
- Polycythaemia.
- Intrapulmonary bleeding (lung haemorrhage) as is seen in Goodpasture's syndrome where the Hb binds the CO.
- Left-to-right shunts (due to increased pulmonary blood flow).

A 28-year-old sales assistant presents to the Accident & Emergency Department with a 10-day history of cough, productive purulent sputum, myalgia, and malaise. Investigations reveal an Hb 9.8 g/dl, reticular sites 4.6%, white cell count 9.0×10^3/l (41% granulocytes, 52% lymphocytes, 4% monocytes), platelets 300×10^3/l, urine dipsticks: blood +++, protein ++, glucose negative, chest X-ray: right lower lobe consolidation.

Question 4 The most likely cause of her symptoms is:

A Mycoplasma pneumonia.
B Haemolytic uremic syndrome.
C Cytomegalovirus infection.
D Staphylococcal pneumonia.
E Tuberculosis.

Question 5 A 50-year-old male has a cavitating lesion on his chest X-ray. The least likely diagnosis is:

A Sarcoidosis.
B Amoebiasis.
C Systemic lupus erythematosus.
D Histoplasmosis.
E Wegener's granulomatosis.

Answer 8

B Hypergammaglobulinaemia is a common feature.

In pulmonary sarcoidosis hypergammaglobulinaemia is common. Berylliosis can produce an identical clinical and histological picture to sarcoidosis. A trans-bronchial biopsy is now the investigation of choice, positive results are seen in 90% of patients with or without X-ray evidence of lung involvement. Of all patients with BHL, 90% show resolution within 2 years. In a minority there is pulmonary infiltration leading to effort dyspnoea, cor pulmonale and death. Chest X-ray in these cases shows mid-zone mottling which may proceed to generalized nodular shadowing. A honeycomb appearance can occasionally occur.

The Kveim test consists of an intradermal injection of sarcoid spleen tissue. If the test is positive, non-caseating granuloma are seen at the injection site in 4–6 weeks, and this finding is highly specific for sarcoid. A negative test does not exclude sarcoid and because of additional risks of infection it is no longer the investigation of choice. Erythema nodosum is associated with a better prognosis.

Chronic berylliosis:
- Hypergammaglobulinaemia.
- Hypercalcuria.
- Hyperuricaemia.
- Polycythaemia.
- 10% cases develop renal calculi.
- Alveolar lavage: increased lymphocytes (CD4 and T-cells)*.
- Diagnosis: by patch test which demonstrates hypersensitivity to beryllium.

*In nonsmokers the intensity of lymphocytosis correlates with clinical severity.

Tutorial

An elevated serum ACE reflects increased macrophage activity which occurs in granulomatous disease and is not specific for sarcoid. It can, however, be used to monitor disease activity once the diagnosis is confirmed.

Causes of increased serum ACE activity include:
Infection:
- TB.
- Leprosy.
- Coccidiomycosis.

Neoplasm:
- Lymphoma.
- Multiple myeloma.

Immunologic:
- Sarcoidosis.
- Extrinsic allergic alveolitis.
- Ulcerative colitis.

Inorganic dust:
- Silicosis.
- Asbestosis.
- Berylliosis.

Metabolic:
- Hyperthyroidism.
- Amyloidosis.
- Gaucher's disease.
- Diabetes mellitus.

Other:
- COPD.
- Osteoarthritis.
- Alcoholic cirrhosis.
- Biliary cirrhosis.
- Familial Mediterranean fever.

Lung function tests in sarcoidosis show:
- Reduction in TLC.
- Reduction in FEV1 and FVC.
- Reduction in TLCO.
- Restrictive lung defect with pulmonary infiltration.

Causes of bilateral hilar lymphadenopathy:
- Sarcoidosis.
- Lymphoma.
- Lymphatic leukaemia.
- Primary TB.
- Mitotic and metastatic disease.
- Acute infections (infectious mononucleosis, whooping cough).

Answer 9

E Scrofula.

A young Afro-Caribbean that presents with systemic disease characterized by a restrictive pulmonary defect, lymphadenopathy, polyarthralgia and hypercalcaemia, is most likely to have sarcoidosis. Sarcoidosis can be complicated by:

- Hypercalcaemia.
- Posterior uveitis.
- Facial nerve palsy.
- Bone cysts.

Scrofula is massive cervical lymph node enlargement seen in TB. Hypercalcaemia is common in sarcoid and is associated with hypercalcuria, which explains the nephrocalcinosis and renal caniculi seen in this condition. The mechanism underlying this is increased circulation and sensitivity to 1,25-dihydroxy vitamin D3 (with 1-alpha hydroxylation occurring in sarcoid macrophages in the lung as well as the normal hydroxylation at the kidney). Phalangeal cysts are common and present with pain and swelling of digits.

Ocular complications of sarcoid:
- Anterior uveitis is more common (red painful eye with misty vision).
- Posterior uveitis is also seen in toxoplasmosis (progressive loss of vision).
- Conjunctivitis.
- Keratoconjunctivitis sicca with lacrymal gland enlargement.

Uveoparotid fever:
- Bilateral uveitis.
- Parotid gland enlargement.
- Facial nerve palsy.

Answer 10

C In foetal haemoglobin.

When the oxygen dissociation curve shifts to the left, the haemoglobin has a greater affinity for oxygen and is less likely to release it. When the curve shifts to the right, oxygen affinity is less and oxygen is released at lower tensions.

Causes of shift to the left:
- Hypothermia.
- Alkalosis.
- Abnormal haemoglobin.
- Foetal haemoglobin.
- Reduced 2,3-DPG (as in following massive blood transfusion).

Causes of shift to the right:
- Chronic increase PCO_2.
- Acidosis.
- Exercise (increased lactate).
- Increased 2,3-DPG.
- Chronic hypoxia (which stimulates increased 2,3-DPG production).

A 48-year-old malt worker presents with breathlessness on exertion and a dry cough. Examination reveals a few aspiratory crackles but no other abnormalities. Investigations: FBC normal, PEFR 550 l/min (predicted 590–650 l/min), FEV1/FVC 78%, O_2 Sat 95% on air, KCO 88%, CXR: miliary shadowing.

Question 11 The most likely diagnosis is:

A Occupational asthma.
B Extrinsic allergic alveolitis.
C Emphysema.
D Allergic bronchopulmonary aspergillosis.
E Chronic bronchitis.

A confused dyspnoeic 60-year-old male is found to have a PaO_2 of 49 mmHg (6.5 kPa) and a PCO_2 of 56 mmHg (7.5 kPa). The Hb is 16.5 g/dl.

Question 12 The following is most likely:

A This abnormality is in keeping with type I respiratory failure.
B He is likely to have central cyanosis.
C Acute pulmonary embolism is a likely diagnosis.
D He has primary polycythaemia.
E These data are consistent with damage of lung tissue.

Answer 11

B Extrinsic allergic alveolitis.

Extrinsic allergic alveolitis is mediated by a type III hypersensitivity reaction based on the precipitin and immune complex formation.

Atopic individuals have type I hypersensitivity. The condition can, however, occur in atopic individuals.

Examples of extrinsic allergic alveolitis include:

Farmer's lung:
- Affects 1/10 working farmers.
- The antigen is thermophilic *Actinomycete microspora faeni.*
- Exposure results from handling mouldy hay and vegetables.

Bird fancier's lung:
- Antigens are found in bird's feathers and excreta (especially pigeons).
- Common in loft cleaners, pigeon farmers.

Malt worker's lung:
- Causative agent is *Aspergillus clavatus.*
- Exposure to germinating barley.

Humidifier fever:
- Caused by a variety of bacteria and amoebae.
- Exposure to contaminated air conditioning and humidifier systems.

Tutorial

Symptoms:
In the exam these may be divided into acute or chronic.

Acute symptoms:
- Occur several hours (usually between 8 and 12) after exposure.
- Fever, malaise, dry cough, SOB.
- Examination shows: fever, tachypnoea, coarse end expiratory crackles, and wheeze throughout the chest; there may be cyanosis, which can be severe and occurs at rest.
- Investigations show: increase in polymorphonuclear count; CXR may show miliary shadowing.

Chronic symptoms:
- Effort dyspnoea.
- Cough.
- Cor pulmonale.
- Cachexia.

Investigations show:
- Restrictive ventilatory defect.
- Reduced gas transfer.
- CXR: fluffy nodular shadows which may progress to honeycomb lung.

Treatment in the early stages is high-dose steroids which may allow for regression. In end stage (established fibrosis), intensive TX plus compensation are offered.

Answer 12

B He is likely to have central cyanosis.

The clinical picture suggests type II respiratory failure. This patient will almost certainly have central cyanosis.

In type II respiratory failure there is a hypoxia accompanied by hypercapnoea. It is due to ventilatory failure and occurs in:
- Chest wall deformities.
- COPD.
- Muscle weakness, e.g. Guillain–Barré syndrome.
- Central respiratory depression.

Type I respiratory failure is characterized by acute hypoxaemia. Carbon dioxide is normal or reduced. It occurs in conditions in which there is damage to lung tissue including:
- Pneumonia.
- ARDS.
- Fibrosing alveolitis.
- Pulmonary oedema.

Question 13 A 50-year-old male is admitted with worsening breathlessness. His chest X-ray shows pleural calcification. The following is unlikely to be the cause of his symptoms:

A Histoplasmosis.
B Haemothorax.
C Tuberculosis.
D Silicosis.
E Asbestosis.

Question 14 Cystic fibrosis is not associated with the following:

A Infertility.
B Complete villous atrophy of the jejunal mucosa.
C Rectal prolapse.
D Gall stones.
E A low concentration of sodium in the sweat.

Question 15 The following statement is false:

A The right hilum is lower than the left.
B The right main bronchus is more vertical than the left.
C The upper zones are less well perfused than middle or lower lobes.
D Lymphatic drainage from the left lung is via the thoracic duct.
E The mean pulmonary artery pressure is 30 mmHg (4 kPa).

Question 16 The following is not true for Legionnaire's disease:

A Bloody diarrhoea is a recognized feature.
B Patients may present with confusion.
C Hypocalcaemia is common.
D Radiological changes may persist for 2 months after the acute illness.
E Rifampicin can be used to treat mild disease.

Answer 13

D Silicosis.

Pleural calcification is seen in tuberculosis and histoplasmosis where it may be extensive. Artificial pneumothorax, which was once used to treat TB, is another cause. Blood in the pleural space can also result in pleural calcification. Asbestosis is often accompanied by the formation of pleural plaques which calcify. Histoplasmosis, chickenpox, and miliary tuberculosis also produce fine nodular calcification known as miliary calcification. Silicosis causes eggshell calcification of enlarged hilar lymph nodes.

Answer 14

E A low concentration of sodium in the sweat.

Tutorial

Inheritance of cystic fibrosis is AR affecting 1/2000 births. Survival to 40+ years is now common, with older patients having an increased risk of cirrhosis. The commonest lung pathogen is *Staphylococcus aureus*. Pseudomonas is more common in adolescence. Twenty percent of patients develop allergic bronchopulmonary aspergillosis.

Patients with cystic fibrosis have infertility problems. Male patients are infertile as a result of absence of the vas deferens. Females have reduced fertility but may conceive. Cystic fibrosis is a recognized cause of malabsorption due to exocrine pancreatic insufficiency, and villous atrophy in the small bowel is well documented.

Symptoms consist of steatorrhoea, failure to thrive, recurrent chest infections, and bronchiectasis due to abnormal mucous production.

Rectal prolapse is a feature as a result of chronic constipation. Meconium ileus occurs in the newborn, and bowel obstruction due to constipation may occur in adults (meconium ileus adult equivalent). There is an increased incidence of cholesterol gall stones and also an increased sodium concentration in the sweat.

Answer 15

E The mean pulmonary artery pressure is 30 mmHg (4 kPa).

The right main bronchus is more vertical than the left, which explains why foreign bodies and aspiration are more common on the right side.

The right hilum lies opposite the 3rd rib and is lower than the left, which lies at the 1st rib. In 90% of patients the right dome of the diaphragm is higher than the left. Hilar shadows are due to pulmonary vessels. The upper zones are less well perfused than middle or lower lobes. Lymphatic drainage from the left lung is via the thoracic duct.

The mean pulmonary pressure in a healthy individual is 15 mmHg (2 kPa).

Answer 16

E Rifampicin can be used to treat mild disease.

Infection with *Legionella pneumophila* usually begins with a high pyrexia, malaise, and myalgia. Gastrointestinal symptoms are common and may precede respiratory symptoms. They consist of nausea, vomiting, abdominal pain, and diarrhoea which may be bloody.

Confusion, delirium, and coma are common in the elderly.

Diagnosis is made by serology or immunofluorescence.

Treatment is with erythromycin with addition of rifampicin in severe cases. In 90% of cases the CXR shows consolidation which is lobar and may be bilateral. Radiological changes may persist for 2 months after the acute illness.

Investigations show:

- Hyponatraemia.
- Hypocalcaemia.
- Hypophosphataemia.
- Hypoalbuminaemia.
- Lymphopenia with neutrophilia are common.
- Renal failure with myoglobinuria may be present.

A 50-year-old publican is referred to the Chest Clinic with malaise, dry cough, and exercise-induced dyspnoea. He smokes 20 cigarettes a day but stopped drinking alcohol 1 year ago when he was found to have chronic hepatitis. On examination he is clubbed with palmer erythema and inspiratory crackles at both lung bases. A high resolution CT scan shows reduced lung volumes, septal thickening, and multiple areas of ground glass change.

Question 17 The following is most likely to be the diagnosis:

A Hypersensitivity pneumonitis.
B Intrinsic allergic alveolitis.
C Systemic lupus with haematosis.
D Emphysema.
E Cryptogenic fibrosing alveolitis.

Question 18 The following statement is not true for primary pulmonary hypertension:

A Is more common in young women.
B May be due to an underlying atrial septal defect.
C Is associated with a prominent a-wave in the jugular venous pressure.
D Peripheral lung fields are plethoric on chest X-ray.
E Patients should be anticoagulated.

Question 19 The following is not true regarding antituberculous medication:

A Red/green colour blindness with ethambutol.
B Pyrazinamide is useful in patients with liver impairment.
C Optic neuritis can be caused by isoniazid.
D Eosinophilia and respiratory symptoms with rifampicin.
E Pyridoxine reduces the incidence of peripheral neuropathy due to isoniazid.

A 33-year-old teacher was admitted from Accident & Emergency with a 1-month history of increasing shortness of breath. She had lost her appetite and 3 kg in weight. She had been treated with two courses of antibiotics from her GP without effect. She had suffered from pneumococcal pneumonia 2 years previously and had been a lifelong nonsmoker. On examination she was febrile and cachexic. There were umbilicated lesions present on her face and hands. Respiratory examination revealed vesicular breath sounds with fine bibasal inspiratory crepitations. Investigations: Hb 10.9 g/dl, WCC 3.9 × 10^9/l, platelets 254 × 10^9/l, sodium 127 mmol/l, potassium 4.3 mmol/l, bicarbonate 26 mmol/l, urea 4.8 mmol/l, creatinine 62 µmol/l, blood gases: pH 7.4, PCO_2 22 mmHg (3 kPa), PO_2 81 mmHg (10.8 kPa), base excess +0.2, saturation 97%, CXR interstitial shadowing across both mid zones with basal and apical sparing and bilateral cyst formation.

Question 20 The most likely diagnosis is:

A Rickettsia.
B Influenza.
C Adenovirus.
D Mycoplasma.
E Psittacosis.

Answer 17

E Cryptogenic fibrosing alveolitis.

The patient has a severe, restrictive lung defect with radiographic evidence of active alveolitis (ground-glass). Cryptogenic fibrosing alveolitis usually presents insidiously in middle-aged men.

Fibrosing alveolitis is common with polyarthritis. Symptoms are a dry, nonproductive, and intractable cough and progressive dyspnoea, progressing to pulmonary hypertension and cor pulmonale.

Rheumatoid factor is positive in 50% of patients. One in ten patients with rheumatoid arthritis have fibrosing alveolitis. ANF is positive in 45% of patients, but manifestations of SLE are rare. The ESR is high. RFTs show a restrictive pattern with reduced gas transfer and hypoxia on blood gases. Broncho-alveolar lavage demonstrates an increase in the neutrophil count.

Signs include clubbing in 70%, cyanosis, and bilateral fine end inspiratory crackles at bases. The CXR has a ground glass appearance progressing to honeycomb.

Tutorial

Associations with fibrosing alveolitis include:
- Scleroderma.
- Sjögren's syndrome.
- Chronic active hepatitis.
- Raynaud's disease.
- Dermatomyositis.
- Coeliac disease.
- Ulcerative colitis.
- Renal tubular acidosis.

Answer 18

D Peripheral lung fields are plethoric on chest X-ray.

Primary pulmonary HT is more common in young women. The aetiology is unknown but it is thought to be due to:
- Recurrent small PEs.
- Pulmonary vasoconstriction.
- Slimming pills (fenfluramine).
- Oral contraceptives.

Other conditions known to produce pulmonary hypertension as a secondary effect are:
- Increased pulmonary blood flow as in left-to-right shunts through VSD, ASD, PDA.
- Increases in the pulmonary venous and capillary pressure occurs in LVF, mitral valve disease, and pulmonary venoocclusive disease, which will result in an elevation of the pulmonary arterial pressure. The pulmonary wedge pressure will be raised in these cases.

Patients should be anticoagulated due to the risks of recurrent pulmonary emboli. Diuretics can be used for right ventricular failure and calcium antagonists are of little use. The most definitive treatment is a heart and lung transplant.

Answer 19

B Pyrazinamide is useful in patients with liver impairment.

Antituberculous medication can have serious side-effects. Ethambutol can cause optic neuritis, red/green colour blindness, and peripheral neuritis. Isoniazid produces a peripheral neuritis which can be prevented by use of pyridoxine. It can also produce an optic neuritis, SLE-like syndrome, pellagra, and Stevens–Johnson syndrome. Rifampicin colours body secretions orange, deranges LFTs, and causes SOB with or without eosinophilia.

Pyrazinamide is contraindicated in liver damage and is hepatotoxic, causing jaundice, hepatomegaly, and liver failure.

Answer 20

D Mycoplasma.

Primary atypical pneumonia may be caused by all the examples except adenovirus.

In mycoplasma infection, the presence of cold agglutinins results in haemolysis. There is often a discrepancy between dramatic changes on the chest X-ray and relative well-being of the patient. Patients respond to macrolide antibiotics,

13 Rheumatology

Question 1 Arthropathy is a recognized feature of all of the following except:

A TB.
B Sarcoidosis.
C Lichen planus.
D Hyperparathyroidism.
E Dermatomyositis.

Question 2 A 35-year-old male presents with a swollen, painful, and erythematous right knee. The following finding would suggest a diagnosis of acute pyogenic arthritis:

A Can be confidently diagnosed by finding a polymorph leucocytosis in the synovial fluid.
B May complicate infection with Brucella species.
C Is rare in patients with rheumatoid arthritis.
D *Staphylococcus aureus* is responsible for 50% of cases.
E The ESR falls more promptly than CRP on treatment.

Question 3 The following conditions are associated with the finding of rheumatoid factor in the serum with the exception of:

A Wegener's granulomatosis.
B Fibrosing alveolitis.
C Malaria.
D Relatives of patients with rheumatoid arthritis.
E Infectious mononucleosis.

Answer 1

C Lichen planus.

Tuberculosis and sarcoidosis are complicated by a mono- or polyarthropathy. Lichen planus does not affect the joints. Osteitis fibrosa et cystica occurs in hyperparathyroidism, affecting most commonly the hands and the pelvis.

Tutorial

Conditions producing primarily monoarthritis:
- Septic arthritis.
- Gout/pseudogout.
- Haemarthrosis.
- Malignancy.

Conditions producing primarily polyarthritis:
- Viral infections, e.g. hepatitis, EBV infection.
- SLE.
- Henoch–Schönlein purpura.
- Stevens–Johnson syndrome.
- Acute rheumatic fever.
- Gonorrhoea.
- Sjögrens syndrome (usually RA picture).
- Ulcerative colitis (mainly joints of lower limbs).
- Dermatomyositis.
- Polymyalgia rheumatica and giant cell arteritis.

Osteoarthritis and spondyloarthritides may produce either picture.

Answer 2

B May complicate infection with Brucella species.

Septic arthritis is caused by haematogenous spread of infective organisms. It may also arise from adjacent sites of osteomyelitis.

Diagnosis is confirmed by demonstrating the presence of organisms in the synovial fluid. Polymorph leucocytes may be raised in other inflammatory states such as the crystal arthropathies, and are hence nonspecific.

Staphylococcus aureus is responsible for 80% of cases. After treatment the CRP falls more rapidly than the ESR.

Tutorial

Patients with underlying joint disease, on steroids, or immunocompromised from other causes are at greater risk. Clinically, the joint is red, hot, very tender, and resists movement. Urgent treatment with antibiotics is mandatory to prevent joint ankyloses and destruction.

Other causes of acute pyogenic arthritis include:
- *Haemophilus influenzae.*
- Gonococcus.
- TB.
- Brucella.
- *Salmonella typhi.*

Answer 3

A Wegener's granulomatosis.

Rheumatoid factor is an autoantibody, usually of the IgM class directed against human IgG. It is found in the serum of patients with joint and connective tissue disease, as well as in some chronic infective states.

Wegener's granulomatosis is associated with a positive ANCA which is present in 95% of patients.

Tutorial

Rheumatoid factor is positive in the following conditions:
- Sjögren's syndrome – 100%.
- Felty's syndrome – 100%.
- Rheumatoid arthritis – 80%.
- SLE – 50%.
- Scleroderma – 30%.
- Mixed connective tissue disorders.
- Infective endocarditis – up to 50%.
- Normal population and relatives of patients with RA – 5–10%.

Low titres of rheumatoid factor are found in:

- TB.
- Leprosy.
- Malaria.
- Viral hepatitis.
- Infectious mononucleosis.
- Elderly patients.
- Chronic active hepatitis (HbsAg negative).
- Fibrosing alveolitis.

Question 4 The following statement is false regarding rheumatoid arthritis:

A Is associated with HLA DR4.
B Palpable splenomegaly occurs in 20% of cases.
C May give rise to a positive Coombs' test.
D Prognosis is particularly poor in patients presenting between 15–30 years of age.
E X-ray of affected joints shows juxta-articular osteoporosis.

A 73-year-old male gives a 4-month history of polyarthralgia, iritis, early morning stiffness lasting for 2 hours, and weight loss. There is synovitis of his left knee and 2nd and 3rd MCP joints on both hands. Blood tests showed Hb 9.0 g/dl, normal MCV, ESR 80 mm/h, CRP 20 mg/l, RF-negative, antinuclear antibody-negative, CK 178 IU/l.

Question 5 The following is true regarding his condition:

A Exudative pleural effusion is a recognized complication.
B Pericardial rub is audible in 30% of patients.
C Optic neuritis may occur.
D Pulmonary eosinophilia is a recognized feature.
E Obliterative bronchiolitis occurs only in smokers.

A 70-year-old female presents with an 8-week history of anorexia and weight loss, headache, pain affecting the cervical and lumbar spine, both shoulders, and hips, early morning stiffness, and low-grade pyrexia (37.5°C [100°F]). Blood tests showed: Hb 8.8 g/dl, normal MCV, CRP 25 mg/l, ESR 86 mm/h, RF-negative, ALP 425 IU/l, and elevated α-1 and α-2 globulins.

Question 6 The most likely diagnosis is:

A Rheumatoid arthritis.
B Temporal arteritis.
C Polymyositis.
D Polymyalgia rheumatica.
E Paraneoplastic syndrome.

Question 7 The following is true of acute gout:

A Does not occur in premenopausal rather than postmenopausal women.
B Commonly occurs in chronic renal failure.
C Crystals are positively birefringent to light.
D Allopurinol is the drug of choice during an acute attack.
E The joint space is frequently reduced on X-ray.

Answer 8

C Familial hypercholesterolaemia.

Gout occurs as a result of hyperuricaemia, although the uric acid does not have to be elevated above normal during an acute attack.

Tutorial

Acute gout may be precipitated by:

- Infection.
- Surgery.
- Starvation.
- Alcoholism.
- Drugs, e.g. thiazide and loop diuretics, low-dose aspirin, ethambutol, and cytotoxics.
- Lead toxicity.
- Primary hyperparathyroidism.
- Hypothyroidism.
- Exercise.

The above conditions are associated with impaired excretion of uric acid. Serum uric acid is also elevated in subjects with hypercholesterolaemia, hypertension, obesity, and high IQ.

Conditions that result in increased production of uric acid:

- Lesch–Nyhan syndrome.
- Glycogen storage diseases, e.g. glucose 6-phosphatase deficiency (type 1).

Myelo- and lymphoproliferative disorders and neoplastic disease are associated with increased purine turnover and affected individuals are more prone to gout.

Answer 9

E Leg ulceration.

There is a close association of giant cell arteritis and PMR, such that they are believed to be variants of the same disease. As a result, patients with cranial arteritis often have symptoms of weight loss, lassitude, and morning stiffness.

Leg ulceration is not a feature.

Tutorial

Symptoms of giant cell arteritis:

- Severe headache with scalp tenderness.
- Blurring vision and even blindness due to involvement of the ophthalmic arteries.
- Jaw claudication.
- Facial pain (due to inflammation of the facial branches of the external carotid).

Complications:

- Amaurosis fugax.
- IIIrd nerve palsy.
- Cortical blindness.
- TIAs.
- Lesions affecting the aorta, renal, coronary, and mesenteric arteries may also occur.

Answer 10

B. Mitral valve prolapse.

Ankylosing spondylitis affects 1/2000 people and presents with morning stiffness affecting the back. It is fourfold more common in males, and 95% of patients are HLA B27-positive.

Complications arise from progressive spinal fusion with sacroiliac involvement causing:

- Fixed kyphotic spine and hyperextended neck.
- Restricted respiratory movement.
- Spontaneous atlanto–axial subluxation and spinal cord damage.

Tutorial

Other complications include:

- Plantar fasciitis.
- Preiostitis of the calcaneum and ischial tuberosities.
- Iritis – 20%.
- Aortic regurgitation, cardiomegaly, and cardiac conduction defects (mitral valve is not affected).
- Amyloidosis.
- Apical lung fibrosis.

Question 11 The following is true of Raynaud's phenomenon:

A It gives rise to pain only when the fingers are white.
B Is a common feature of polyarteritis nodosa.
C May lead to gangrene.
D Is a special risk in workers using vibrating tools.
E Is a recognized finding in carcinoid syndrome.

Question 12 Characteristic features of polyarteritis nodosa include the following with the exception of:

A Renal involvement in 80% of cases.
B Aneurysm formation of the medium sized arteries.
C Eosinophilia.
D Pericarditis.
E Abnormal C3 complement levels.

A 30-year-old male presents with a painful, swollen, right knee, swollen ankles, acutely inflamed eyes, and dysuria. He was previously well except for an episode of gastroenteritis 2 weeks previously. He is HLA-B27 positive.

Question 13 The following statement is true regarding his condition:

A He has a seropositive arthritis.
B He may develop aphthous ulcers as a result of this condition.
C Arthropathy, associated with the finding of Peking cells in the synovial fluid.
D A male to female ratio of 3:1.
E It is not associated with iritis.

Answer 11

C May lead to gangrene.

Raynaud's disease is common affecting 5% of the population. The disorder is bilateral, affecting the fingers more than the toes.

Symptoms are associated with a change in blood flow to the digits:
- Phase 1 – vasoconstriction = pallor.
- Phase 2 – cyanosis.
- Phase 3 – hyperaemia = redness and pain.

Between attacks the digits and pulses are normal. Attacks may last for hours, and result in trophic changes with areas of gangrene. It is more common in people who work with hands immersed in cold water and vibrating tools.

Raynaud's disease may be a feature of connective tissue disease, especially scleroderma, SLE, and rheumatoid arthritis. PAN is associated with skin ulcers and digital vasculitis, but in Raynaud's these are uncommon.

Other causes of Raynaud's phenomenon:
- Drugs (beta-blockers, ergot derivatives).
- Cryoglobinaemia.
- Atherosclerosis, Bueger's disease.
- Thoracic outlet obstruction.
- Polycythaemia, leukaemia.
- Amyloidosis.
- Trauma.

Answer 12

E Abnormal C3 complement levels.

PAN is relatively unique in connective tissue disease in that it is more common in men.

Tutorial

Pathology: fibrinoid necrosis and microaneurysm formation, affecting small and medium sized vessels.

Features:
- Fever, malaise, myalgia, arthralgia.
- Hypertension – 50%. Sometimes malignant.
- Renal impairment – 80%. Acute nephritic/nephrotic syndrome, progressive renal failure.
- Cardiac – 70%. Myocardial ischaemia, arrhythmia, pericarditis, heart failure.
- CNS – 50%. Peripheral neuropathy, mononeuritis multiplex, SAH.
- GIT – 50%. Abdominal pain, bowel/hepatobiliary infarction.
- Respiratory – 40%. Churg–Strauss syndrome (asthma with pulmonary eosinophilia).
- Skin – 25%. Arteritic lesions, tender subcutaneous.
- Joints – 10%. Nondeforming polyarthritis, mainly of the lower limbs.

Investigations show:
- Increased ESR.
- pANCA in microscopic PAN against myeloperoxidase (cANCA against protease 3 is seen in Wegener's granulomatosis).
- Neutrophil leucocytosis (reflects the severity of the disease and can be used to monitor the response to therapy).
- Eosinophilia.
- Hepatitis B surface antigen is positive in 30%.
- Platelets and complement are usually normal.

Answer 13

C Arthropathy, associated with the finding of Peking cells in the synovial fluid.

This clinical scenarion satisfies the diagnostic criteria for Reiter's syndrome.

Reiter's syndrome cosists of a triad of:
- Conjunctivitis.
- Nonspecific urethritis.
- Seronegative arthritis.

Tutorial

Reiter's syndrome may occur in two main situations:
1. Postvenereal infection.
2. Following GI infection with:
- Shigella.
- Campylobacter.
- Salmonella.
- Yersinia.

It is 20-fold more common in males aged 15–35 years. HLA B27 is positive in 80%.

Other features include:

- Arthritis (symmetrical involvement of the knees, ankles, and feet).
- Sacroiliitis.
- Achilles tendonitis.
- Plantar fasciitis.
- Iritis.
- Keratoderma blenorragica.
- Mouth ulcers.
- Circinate balanitis (painless serpiginous rash).
- Aortic incompetence.
- Nail dystrophy.
- Pleurisy.
- Peripheral neuropathy.

Peking cells are neutrophils containing macrophages. X-rays may reveal periostitis at ligament insertions and rheumatoid-like changes.

A 40-year-old female presents with an 8-month history of erythematous rash over the knuckles, elbows, and eyelids, with no response to topical steroids. She subsequently noticed stiffness and soreness of her shoulders and proximal legs. She has weakness with difficulty lifting heavy objects or rising from a squatting position. The CK was elevated at 5130 IU/l.

Question 14 The following statement is not true regarding her condition:

A May be associated with carcinoma of the ovary.
B Arthropathy particularly affects the small joints of the hands.
C Spontaneous fibrillation on EMG is characteristic.
D The WCC is normal during acute episodes.
E Dysphagia occurs in 5%.

Question 15 A 35-year-old female with SLE gave birth to a child who was found to have congenital heart block. The following antibodies will be positive in the maternal serum:

A Anti-SM.
B Anti-Ro.
C Anti-Jo-1.
D Anti-La.
E Anti-RNP.

A 37-year-old West Indian male is admitted to hospital with a 3-month history of progressive dyspnoea and a nonproductive cough. He had complained that his fingers became very painful and pale in the cold weather. On examination abnormal findings were confined to the hands where the skin was tight and shiny, and the chest where there were fine crepitations at the bases. Investigations: Hb, WCC, ESR normal. CXR: patchy shadowing in both midzones and bases.

Question 16 The likely diagnosis is:

A MCTD.
B Systemic sclerosis.
C Limited cutaneous scleroderma.
D SLE.
E Behçet's disease.

Answer 14

D. The WCC is normal during acute episodes.

Dermatomyositis has an association with underlying malignancy. This is most frequently bronchial carcinoma in males and ovarian carcinoma in females.

Tutorial

Features:
- Muscle pain and tenderness – 50%.
- Arthritis – 50% (may resemble rheumatoid arthritis).
- Dysphagia – 50% (oesophageal muscle involvement).
- Raynaud's phenomenon.
- Sjögren's syndrome.

Investigations show:
- Muscle enzymes – CK and aldolase are raised and can be used to monitor treatment.
- EMG – short polyphasic motor potentials with spontaneous fibrillation.
- Muscle biopsy – necrosis and disruption of fibres with fibrosis.
- Positive ANF and RF.
- Increased WCC and ESR.

Answer 15

B. Anti-Ro.

Anti-Ro antibodies in the maternal serum may cause foetal congenital heart block. Anti-Jo-1 antibodies are seen in 30% of patients with polymyositis. Anti-RNP occur in 25% of patients with SLE, and less frequently in systemic sclerosis and polymyositis. High titres are found in mixed connective tissue disease.

Anticentromere antibodies occur in CREST.

Answer 16

B. Systemic sclerosis.

In patients with systemic sclerosis, dysphagia is common, occurring in 65% of patients. Antibodies to SC 70 are seen in 25% of patients and are directed against topoisomerase-1 which is a DNA charging enzyme. LE cells are present in 10% of patients, ANF is positive in 80%, and anticentromere antibodies are present in CREST.

Steatorrhoea and malabsorption are rare. There is no evidence that immunosuppressive drugs significantly retard disease expression.

Tutorial

System involvement in systemic sclerosis:

Renal:
- Progressive renal failure – 20%.
- Hypertension is usually late and often malignant.

Respiratory:
- Diffuse interstitial fibrosis.
- Aspiration pneumonitis from oesophageal motility disorder.

Cardiac:
- Cardiomyopathy.
- CCF.
- Pericardial effusion.

Skin: (75%)
- Raynaud's, sclerodactyly, telangiectasia.
- Nonpitting oedema of distal extremities.
- Vitiligo and skin pigmentation – 50%.
- Sicca syndrome – 5%.
- Morphoea (benign and rarely proceeds to systemic sclerosis).

Question 17 Synovial fluid from a normal joint has all the following except:

A A high viscosity.
B Glucose level half that of blood.
C Cell count of $<0.2 \times 10^9$/l.
D The presence of a fibrin clot.
E A few crystals of hydroxyapatite.

A 28-year-old previously fit and well female presents with a swollen painful right calf. On examination livedo reticularis is present in both legs and her right calf is swollen. Blood tests showed WCC 5.8×10^9/l (lymphocytes 1.5×10^9/l, neutrophils 3.3×10^9/l), platelets 86×10^9/l, ESR 10 mm/h, and CRP 5 mg/l.

Question 18 The following is not true of her condition:

A Antibodies are directed against cardiolipin.
B Thrombocytosis results in thrombo-embolic phenomena.
C False positive VDRL test is recognized.
D May complicate HIV infection.
E Livedo reticularis is a cutaneous manifestation.

A 45-year-old female presents with red eyes, a purpuric rash on both legs, and polyarthralgia affecting the small joints of both hands. Blood tests showed RF >1:5,000, antinuclear antibodies 1:620, anti-ds DNA 1:10, anti-Ro antibodies 1:320, anti-La antibodies 1:320. Hand X-ray showed normal bone density with no erosions.

Question 19 The following is not true of this condition:

A Is more common in women.
B Shirmir's test is indicative if 15 mm of filter paper is not wet within 2 minutes.
C Anti-Ro antibodies occur in 60%.
D May complicate graft-versus-host disease.
E Is associated with hypergammaglobulinaemia.

Question 20 The following is not true regarding cryoglobinaemia:

A Is a rare cause of Raynaud's phenomenon.
B May occur in syphilis.
C Is typically associated with low C4 and C3 levels.
D May complicate myeloma.
E Can make cardiac surgery potentially hazardous.

Answer 17

E. A few crystals of hydroxyapatite.

- Normal synovial fluid is clear and viscous.
- Viscosity is reduced in septic and rheumatoid arthritis, and is very low in gout and pyrophosphate arthropathy.
- The cell count is $<0.2 \times 10^9$/l of mononuclear cells.
- Neutrophils in the synovial fluid indicate infection or inflammation.
- Normal synovial fluid does not contain fibrinogen and crystals are not normally present.

Answer 18

B. Thrombocytosis results in thrombo-embolic phenomena.

The most likely diagnosis with the above clinical features is antiphospholipid syndrome.

The antiphospholipid syndrome is made up of a number of antibodies, including those directed at cardiolipin, antibodies which cause a positive lupus anticoagulant, and antibodies which cause a positive VDRL test for syphilis.

Although thromboembolic disease (venous and arterial) is a common manifestation, thrombocytopenia is characteristic, as opposed to thrombocytosis. Spontaneous and recurrent abortion occurs due to thrombosis of the placental vasculature. Livedo reticularis is a recognized cutaneous manifestation.

The syndrome can occur alone, with SLE, and as a complication of HIV infection. Other rheumatological conditions associated with HIV include polymyositis, Sjögren's syndrome, and necrotizing vasculitis.

Answer 19

B. Shirmir's test is indicative if 15 mm of filter paper is not wet within 2 minutes.

The positive autoantibodies (>1:80) indicate an autoimmune disease. The absence of double-stranded DNA antibodies makes SLE unlikely. The normal hand X-ray does exclude RA, but the presence of Ro and La antibodies suggest primary Sjögren's syndrome.

Sjögren's syndrome is ninefold commoner in women. It is a disease characterized by inflammation and destruction of exocrine glands including:

- Lacrimal (dry eyes).
- Salivary (xerostomia).
- Sweat glands.
- Mucous glands of the bowel, vagina, and bronchial tree, causing constipation and dyspareunia.

In Shirmir's test a piece of filter paper is placed under the lower eyelid. The test is diagnostic if <15 mm is wet within 5 minutes. Lip biopsy is also useful for diagnosis, and shows a mononuclear infiltration (90% CD4 T-cells and 10% B-cells).

Antibodies to ribonucleoprotein are common in primary Sjögren's (anti-Ro – 60%, anti-La – 50%). Sjögren's is associated with HLA DR3, B8, and DQ2.

Answer 20

C. Is typically associated with low C4 and C3 levels.

Cryoglobinaemia may occur in a number of conditions. The most important for the exam are:

- CTD (RA, SLE, Sjögren's).
- Infection (bacterial endocarditis, syphilis, CMV and EBV infection, leprosy).
- Haematological (myeloma, Waldenstrom's macroglobinaemia, myeloproliferative disorders).
- Myocardial infarction, glomerulonephritis.

Cryoglobinaemia is a rare cause of Raynaud's.

14 Mock Examination

Question 1 The following is inconsistent with a compressive lesion at the optic chiasm:

A Left homonymous hemianopia.
B Central field defect.
C Bitemporal hemianopia.
D Right upper homonymous quadrantanopia.
E Right achromatopsia.

Question 2 Muscle atrophy is not a characteristic feature in:

A Cushing's disease.
B Cervical spondylosis.
C Duchenne muscular dystrophy.
D Motor neurone disease.
E Right parietal lobe infarction.

Question 3 The following are all features of Friedreich's ataxia except:

A Peripheral neuropathy.
B Optic atrophy.
C Tremor.
D Stamping gait.
E Restrictive cardiomyopathy.

Question 4 The following is not a feature of an intracranial metastatic tumour:

A Early morning headache.
B Vomiting.
C Epilepsy.
D Impaired upward gaze.
E Monoparesis.

Answer 1

E Right achromatopsia.

Compressive lesions at the optic chiasm most commonly cause a quadrantanopic field defect. Occasionally asymmetrical compression of the chiasm may cause a homonymous defect and, most infrequently, is the only site along the visual pathway to produce a bitemporal hemianopia. Central field defects occur as a result of optic nerve defects or, rarely, with occipital lobe pathology (Anton's syndrome). Anopia is complete loss of vision in one eye.

Tutorial

Knowledge of the anatomical visual pathway and the clinical manifestations of lesions occurring at the various points is necessary; in particular the ability to distinguish clinically between pre- and retrochiasmal lesions (homonymous).

Achromatopsia is an inability to distinguish colours and is due to a bilateral visual processing disorder (in the secondary visual cortex).

Answer 2

E Right parietal lobe infarction.

Muscle atrophy is a prominent feature of lower motor neurone syndromes. The site of pathology may be anywhere from the motor nucleus (anterior horn cell), the motor nerve (anterior) rootlet, the peripheral nerve, to the neuromuscular junction. Muscle atrophy, although not characteristic of myasthenia gravis, does occur. For all practical purposes, marked wasting and atrophy should prompt the diagnosis of the myasthenic syndrome rather than MG. Proximal myopathy is a feature of Cushing's syndrome and of Duchenne's muscular dystrophy where Gower's sign (rising from the floor, having to push with the hands against shins, knees and thighs to reach a standing position) is often seen. Cervical spondylosis can cause focal muscle atrophy in the distribution of the compressed nerve root, although the usual symptoms are those of dysaethesiae.

Tutorial

The question requires an understanding of the motor axis and the essential differences between motor deficits resulting from an UMN and a LMN.

Anterior horn cell diseases: motor neurone disease, poliomyelitis, spinal muscular atrophy (genetic).

Answer 3

E Restrictive cardiomyopathy.

Friedreich's ataxia is a trinucleotide repeat, AR disorder, in which there is spinocerebellar degeneration (tremor) with peripheral neuropathy. The stamping gait is a sign of involvement of the posterior columns in the spinal cord. There is associated optic atrophy and often, in the absence of the neuropathy, the young are misdiagnosed with demyelinating disease. There is accompanying retinitis pigmentosa (night blindness). Death is usually a consequence of heart failure from hypertrophic cardiomyopathy. Ichthyosis is a feature of occult malignancy and also Refsum's disease, and its presence helps to differentiate this condition from Friedreich's ataxia.

Tutorial

Knowledge of the main features of Friedreich's ataxia is required, particularly as it is often in the differential diagnosis of many neurological conditions affecting the young.

Trinucleotide repeat diseases: Fragile X syndrome, dystrophia myotonica, Huntington's disease, spinocerebellar ataxia.

Answer 4

C Epilepsy.

The early morning headache occurs because of cerebral vasodilatation, secondary to nocturnal hypoventilation causing hypercapnia. The reduced compliance of the brain in the presence of tumour does not allow for compensation in ICP. Vomiting is typically not accompanied by nausea. Impaired upward gaze is a feature of midbrain compression (especially in acute hydrocephalus). Monoparesis results from deposits in the motor strip, internal capsule, cerebral peduncles, or brainstem Epilepsy is an idiopathic seizure disorder.

Tutorial

Recognition of the physiological response to intracranial hypertension, and the clinical manifestations is required.

Question 5 Features of a left ulnar nerve lesion below the elbow include all the following except:

A Wasting of the thenar eminence.
B Wasting of the hypothenar eminence.
C Erb's sign.
D Altered sensation on the inner aspect of the ring finger.
E Claw hand deformity.

Question 6 The investigation least useful in the diagnosis of myasthenia gravis is:

A Acetylcholine receptor antibodies.
B Edrophonium stimulation test.
C PEFR.
D Single fibre EMG.
E CT scan of the chest.

Question 7 The treatment least useful in the management of alcohol abuse is:

A Chlordiazopoxide.
B Diazepam.
C Thiamine.
D Disulfiram.
E Lactulose.

Question 8 The following conditions are associated with the presence of *café-au-lait* spots except:

A Neurofibromatosis type II.
B von Recklinghausen's disease.
C Multiple endocrine neoplasia type I.
D Tuberous sclerosis.
E von Hippel–Lindau syndrome.

Question 9 All of the below conditions can be inherited in an autosomal dominant fashion with the exception of:

A Friedreich's ataxia.
B Motor neurone disease.
C Alzheimer's disease.
D Neurofibromatosis type II.
E Myotonic dystrophy.

Answer 5

A Wasting of the thenar eminence.

The ulnar nerve orginates from the medial cord of the brachial plexus (the predominant input from C8/T1 roots). Lesions below the elbow spare the branches to the ulnar half of flexor digitorum profundus and thus flexion at the DIPJ is preserved, producing the characteristic claw hand deformity. Ulnar nerve lesions will result in wasting of the hypothenar eminence, whether above or below the elbow. The sensory distribution includes the ulnar aspect of the ring finger and the little finger. The thenar eminence is supplied by the median nerve. Erb described the 'waiter's tip' sign in a cohort of patients with a brachial plexus injury of the lower roots.

Tutorial

Knowledge of the anatomical course of the ulnar nerve allows the clinical examination to determine the level of the peripheral nerve lesion. The principle here is that the clinical findings on examination can often point to the site of the lesion.

Answer 6

C PEFR.

The modern day diagnosis of myasthenia gravis depends on the finding of fatiguability on single fibre EMG (ocular muscles) and seropositivity for acetylcholine receptor antibodies. The former gold standard, edrophonium stimulation, is now out of favour due to the potential life threatening sequelae and the need to perform it with intubation facilities to hand. Vital capacity is the bedside test of choice for monitoring diaphragmatic function. (PEFR is a more useful test of obstructive airways disease)

Tutorial

Modern day diagnosis of this condition is multispectral. Greater priority should be afforded to minimally invasive tests.

Associations with MG include thymoma (female >male), antiacetylcholine receptor antibodies (80–90% of patients with MG).

Answer 7

E Lactulose.

Disulfiram is used occasionally as a deterrent in patients with alcohol abuse, as it interacts with ethanol to produce a bad hangover effect (also produced with metronidazole). Lactulose is used in the management of alcoholic liver failure as a means of bacterial clearance, and not in the management of ethanol abuse.

Chlordiazopoxide (Librium) and diazepam have a longer half-life than alcohol and interact at the same CNS receptor. They can be used in a reducing regimen to wean patients off the addiction slowly, but are only temporary measures. Thiamine is given to replenish stores which are often depleted in these patients, in order to reduce the likelihood of Wernicke's encephalopathy.

- Wernicke's encephalopathy: ophthalmoplegia, gait disturbance, short-term memory impairment.
- Korsakoff's psychosis: confabulation, hallucinations (mainly visual), occasional paranoia.

Tutorial

Prioritizing the various management strategies is important; treatment of the effects of abuse being paramount to attempts at deterrence.

Answer 8

C Multiple endocrine neoplasia type I.

The presence of six or more *café-au-lait* spots, ≥2 cm is said to be diagnostic of NF I (von Recklinghausen's disease). They are however, seen in the other phakomatoses (von Hippel–Lindau syndrome), NF II and tuberous sclerosis, and MEN IIb.

- von Hippel–Lindau syndrome: autosomal recessive, chromosome 5. Features include cerebellar, renal, and spinal haemangioblastomas and retinal tumours.

Tutorial

These skin pigments are found in other neurogenetic conditions, and are not pathognomic.

Answer 9

A Friedreich's ataxia.

There is an inherited form of Alzheimer's disease, which is associated with autosomal dominant inheritance (presenilin genes). The inherited form of MND may be X-linked or AD. Friedreich's ataxia is inherited in a recessive manner.

Tutorial

Many neurological conditions follow defined patterns of inheritance and examples of a few commonly found in exam papers should be revised. Inherited neurological disorders: neurofibromatosis I (AD), myotonic dystrophy (AD), Huntington's disease (AD), Duchenne muscular dystrophy (XR).

NF II: bilateral (occasionally only unilateral) vestibular schwannomas, peripheral plexiform neurofibromata, spinal schwannomas. This is an autosomal dominant condition, chromosome 22. Less than 5% of lesions undergo malignant transformation.

Question 10 The following statement regarding immunoglobulins is not true:

A IgM is the primary mediator of innate immunity.
B IgD is a deficient immunoglobulin and requires IgG to be functional.
C IgA deficiency predisposes to *Neisseria* infection.
D Each immunoglobulin has two epitope binding sites.
E IgM is complement activating.

Question 11 The following statement regarding complement factors is true:

A C2a is the active moiety.
B There is a predisposition to SLE in C3 deficiency.
C There are reduced levels of C3 in C_1esterase deficiency.
D They have binding sites on the surface of lymphocytes.
E Lack of the terminal complex predisposes to bleeding tendency.

Question 12 T-lymphocytes are best described by:

A Are derived from the bone marrow.
B May be classified according to differing cytokine profiles.
C CD8+ T-lymphocytes allow intracellular entry of HIV.
D Are the mediators of hyperacute rejection following organ transplantation.
E Specificity is governed by genes on chromosome 3.

Question 13 The following statement regarding hypersensitivity is true:

A Type IV is the predominant mechanism in early asthma.
B Type III involves cytotoxic antibodies.
C There is absent type IV hypersensitivity in *Mycobacteria leprae* infection.
D Graves' disease is caused by the action of a blocking autoantibody.
E The cause of farmer's lung is a type III reaction.

Answer 10

A IgM is the primary mediator of innate immunity.

IgM is the primary antibody produced during a challenge. Subsequently, on repeated exposure IgG is produced by plasma cells, after undergoing class switching in the lymph node germinal centre. IgA is the predominant antibody at mucosal surfaces and a deficiency makes STD more likely. IgM immune complex is the activator of the complement pathway. IgD is an incomplete immunoglobulin and requires IgG to be functionally active. Each immunoglobulin has two antigen–epitope binding sites, made up of both light and heavy chain components.

Tutorial

A basic knowledge of the immunological response and the role of the various antibodies is required.

Primary immunodeficiencies include Bruton's (hypogammaglobulinaemia), ataxiatelangiectasia (T-cell), common variable immunodeficiency, selective hypo-IgA deficiency (commonest, approximately 1:800 prevalence).

Answer 11

B There is a predisposition to SLE in C3 deficiency.

Factor C3b is the most active factor in the complement cascade, and is the chief opsonin. The C2a4a complex is the activating complex, which itself is formed by the $C1_{qrs}$ complex. Deficiency of C3 predisposes to SLE, whilst those of factors VII, VIII, and IX (terminal complex) predispose to Gram-negative sepsis from *Neiserria* spp..

C_1-esterase deficiency results in reduced levels of C4 (and C2). Complement receptors can be found on NK cells and neutrophils. Deficiency of the DAF forms the basis of PNH.

Tutorial

A basic knowledge of the components of the innate immune system and the clinical effects that result from inherited and acquired deficiencies is required. The terminal components of the pathway form the MAC. An absence of DAF results in the clinical picture of PNH.

Answer 12

B May be classified according to differing cytokine profiles.

T-lymphocytes are derived from the thymus and are subdivided by CD8/4+ surface antigen, and further classified into $TH_{1/2}$ by cytokine profiles. CD4+ cells are the entry points for HIV virus, along with co-factor, the chemokine receptor 5. Hyperacute rejection is mediated by preformed antibodies, whilst acute rejection is thought to be mediated by cytotoxic T-cells. T-cell specificity is determined by a gene in the major histocompatibility complex on chromosome 6.

Tutorial

The origin of T-cells should be revised and the differences that characterize them (surface markers, cytokine profiles).

Cytokine profiles: Th_1: IL-1, IFN-γ, IL-2; Th_2: IL-8, IL-12.

Answer 13

E The cause of farmer's lung is a type III reaction.

Traditionally, there have been four types of hypersensitivity reaction. Type I is IgE mediated and relates to presensitization. Type II, as seen in Graves' disease, is due to cytotoxic antibodies. Type III, serum sickness, is immune complex mediated and requires complement activation (e.g. farmer's lung). Type IV is seen in tuberculosis, and is termed delayed hypersensitivity and is typified by the Heaf test. The response is impaired but not absent in leprosy.

Tutorial

The clinical manifestations of the hypersensitivity syndromes should be understood to appreciate how the immune system can go wrong.

Asthma results initially from a type I reaction and subsequently from a type IV process.

Question 14 The following are recognized autoimmune disorders with the exception of:

A Hypoparathyroidism.
B Hyperthyroidism.
C Crohn's disease.
D Pemphigus vulgaris.
E Coeliac disease.

Question 15 Rheumatoid factor is best described by:

A Is most commonly IgG anti-IgM.
B Forms cryoglobulins at room temperature.
C Is found in 95% of patients with rheumatoid arthritis.
D Does not bind complement factors avidly.
E Is almost always deposited in the kidney.

Question 16 The following statement regarding T-helper cells is not true:

A Have MHC class I restriction.
B TH_1-cells produce IFN-γ.
C Lacking a cofactor on the surface, are immune from HIV infection.
D Orchestrate the antibody response.
E Have dimeric receptors.

Question 17 The following statements on chronic myeloid leukaemia are all not true, except:

A There is an associated chromosomal duplication.
B Basophilia is an uncommon finding.
C Is a cause of secondary polycythaemia.
D Has a poor prognosis, even in the early stages.
E Bone marrow transplantation has not been shown to be of benefit.

Question 18 Acute myeloid leukaemia is characterized by all of the following, except:

A Peak incidence in the young.
B Higher incidence in men than women.
C The presence of chromosomal translocation.
D Nuclear inclusion bodies.
E An associated clotting abnormality.

Answer 14

C Crohn's disease.

Autoimmune hypoparathyroidism forms part of polyglandular syndrome type I, which has a genetic basis. Coeliac disease is associated with antitransglutamase antibodies. The association between Crohn's disease and *Mycobacteria paratuberculosis* is very tentative and not universally accepted. Graves' hyperthyroidism is associated with an activating autoantibody that increases intracellular signal transduction.

Tutorial

Knowledge of the clinically important autoimmune syndromes is required.

Syndromes include: Goodpasture's syndrome, pemphigus vulgaris, Addison's disease, myasthenia gravis, Graves' disease, Hashimoto's thyroiditis.

Answer 15

A Is most commonly IgG anti-IgM.

Rheumatoid factor is most commonly IgG against IgM, and is found in approximately 60% of patients with RA and 5% of the elderly population. Cryoglobulins form at below room temperature; they are 'cold' haemaglutinins. Rheumatoid factor, an immune complex, binds C3 avidly. Rheumatoid factor circulates in the serum and only a small proportion is found in the kidney. The kidney is not heavily involved in rheumatoid disease.

Tutorial

A finding of rheumatoid factor seropositivity is useful. Seropositivity is associated with a worse prognosis, and nodular disease.

Answer 16

A Have MHC class I restriction.

T-cells express a dimeric receptor on their surface within which antigen epitopes are presented; they are usually composed of $\alpha\beta$ subunits. T-helper cells are class II restricted, a molecule which is present only on antigen presenting cells, unlike MHC I molecules which are present on all nucleated cells. The coreceptor for HIV on CD4 cells is thought to be CRC-4 (chemokine receptor). The TH_1 subpopulation produces mainly IFN-γ, and IL-1. The chemokine receptor-4 serves as a coreceptor for HIV entry into CD4+ cells. There is a well published series of a family of sex workers in East Africa who are free of HIV and AIDS, in whom immunophenotyping has revealed a lack of CRC-5.

Tutorial

Different clinical syndromes may result from a differing T-cell response. Subsets of T-helper cells exist that modulate these responses.

Mycobacterium leprae: tuberculoid form (Th_1) is less contagious; lepromatous form (Th_2) is highly contagious.

Answer 17

C Is a cause of secondary polycythaemia.

Chronic myeloid leukaemia, is one of the four recognized myeloproliferative disorders, and in common with the others, features include raised WCC, platelets, and red cell numbers. They are all associated with splenomegaly and transformation in the late phase to an acute myeloid leukaemia. CML is associated with a characteristic chromosomal translocation (t 9:22 Philadelphia chromosome) and peripheral basophilia. CML generally has a favourable prognosis in the early phase, particularly as sibling bone marrow allografts are being used more as first line therapy.

Tutorial

CML should be studied to appreciate the overlap in clinical and laboratory findings that exists in the myeloproliferative group of disorders. Additionally, to appreciate that genetic mutations underpin haematological as well as solid tumours.

Myleoproliferative disorders: polycythaemia rubra vera, essential thrombocythaemia, myelofibrosis. These may all develop blast crisis, when the prognosis is worse than for AML from the outset. Recent advances have paved the way for a biochemical treatment, designed to antagonize the constitutive activity of the tyrosine kinase receptor that occurs as a result of the Philadelphia mutation.

Answer 18

D Nuclear inclusion bodies.

Acute myeloid leukaemia is an aggressive form of leukaemia that affects young adults. Males are affected more than females. There are characteristic cytoplasmic inclusion bodies, called Auer rods, which help to differentiate from acute lymphoid leukaemia morphologically. Acute promyelocytic leukaemia is associated with DIC. The chromosomal abnormality associated with AML is a translocation (t 15:17).

Tutorial

The clinical and laboratory features of AML should be recognized. AML may be treated with *All*-trans-retinoic acid, or in certain circumstances, allograft bone marrow transplantation.

Question 19 The following are features of multiple myeloma with the exception of:

A Bony pain.
B Normocytic anaemia.
C Renal impairment.
D Autonomic neuropathy.
E Hypercellular marrow aspirate.

Question 20 Cryoglobulins have been found in all of the following conditions except:

A Rheumatoid arthritis.
B Hodgkin's lymphoma.
C SLE.
D Multiple myeloma.
E Hepatitis B infection.

Question 21 Haemophilia A is not characterized by:

A A compensatory increase in Factor IX levels.
B Prolongation of the prothrombin time.
C Low platelet levels.
D Recurrent haemarthrosis.
E Antibodies to Factor VIII.

Question 22 Target cells are not seen in:

A Sickle cell disease.
B Beta-thalassaemia.
C Chronic liver disease.
D Sickle cell trait.
E Abetalipoproteinaemia.

Answer 19

E Hypercellular marrow aspirate.

Myeloma is a malignant transformation of bone marrow plasma cells. It may or may not be associated with a serum paraprotein and urinary light chains. Characteristically there is renal impairment. Autonomic neuropathy may be due to either paraprotein neuropathy or (more commonly) amyloid changes. Diagnosis should not rely on bone marrow aspirate, as this may be normal, and usually requires a trephine biopsy to identify the myeloma cells. A dry marrow aspirate is associated with myelofibrosis. Bony pain is due to bone destruction. A normocytic, normochromic anaemia signifies anaemia of chronic disease.

Tutorial

Myeloma should be studied in great depth in view of the vast number of clinical syndromes that it presents with and the strong association with amyloidosis.

Amyloid is usually AL type in association with myeloma; it is confirmed by finding positive apple-green birefringence on microscopy of tissue (marrow, renal). Rectal biopsy yields positivity in approximately 60% of cases of AA (inflammatory) amyloid. Diagnosis is supplemented by performing a SAP scan.

Answer 20

B Hodgkin's lymphoma.

Cryoglobulins are serum proteins that precipitate at low temperature. They are associated with a number of conditions, and are classified according to composition (e.g. rheumatoid factor, paraproteins). They may form immune complexes and if precipitated can cause hyperviscosity sequelae. Hodgkin's disease is associated with warm haemaglutinin antibodies. Myeloma, rheumatoid disease, SLE, and chronic hepatitis B infection are all associated with cryoglobulins.

Tutorial

A knowledge of the different forms of cryoglobulins is required and the array of associated clinical syndromes with which they feature.

Warm antibodies: can be associated with autoimmune haemolytic anaemia or Hodgkin's disease.

Answer 21

C Low platelet levels.

Haemophilia A is an inherited X-linked recessive disorder characterized by spontaneous or minor traumatic haemarthroses. There is characteristic prolongation of the APTT only. Compensatory mechanisms cause an elevation of the factor IX level. Antibodies to factor VIII develop with prolonged therapy with recombinant factor VIII injections. von Willebrand's disease is associated with recurrent epistaxis and prolonged APTT.

Tutorial

An in depth knowledge of this common X-linked inherited condition is necessary; this includes the laboratory investigations that help differentiate it from other conditions, e.g. lupus anticoagulant.

Prolonged APTT is found in unfractionated heparin therapy, lupus anticoagulant, factor VIII and IX deficiencies, and von Willebrand factor deficiency. Correction of the APTT with normal serum is suggestive of deficiency, whereas failure to correct the APTT suggests the presence of an inhibitor.

Answer 22

E Abetalipoproteinaemia.

Target cells are red cells with central staining and a peripheral rim of pallor (also described as Mexican hat cells). They are most commonly seen in chronic ethanolic liver disease and iron deficiency anaemia. However, they may also be seen in HbSC, and thalassaemia.

Tutorial

Students should appreciate that target cells feature in blood films from patients with an array of medical conditions, and that they are by no means pathognomic. A large number of target cells on the blood film of a patient with HbSS, should raised the possibility of HbSC disease.

Conditions in which target cells are seen include: chronic liver disease, folate deficiency, haemoglobinopathies.

Question 23 Multiple myeloma is often associated with all of the following except:

A Osteoclastic bone lesions.
B Raised ALP.
C Plasma cells in the bone marrow.
D No serum paraprotein.
E An interstitial pneumonitis.

Question 24 The following are not features of infectious mononucleosis:

A Warm haemagglutinin disease.
B Antibodies to Epstein–Barr virus.
C Abnormal T-lymphocytes.
D Red cell agglutination.
E High MCV.

Question 25 The following is true of sickle cell disease:

A Sickle cells present on the blood film only in states of anoxia.
B Aplastic crisis is usually precipitated by Coxsackie virus.
C Proctitis in childhood.
D Predisposition to infection from encapsulated bacteria.
E Hypersplenism in adulthood.

Question 26 The following are all causes of a positive direct Coombs' test with the exception of:

A Chronic treatment with methyldopa.
B Acute transfusion reaction.
C Haemorrhagic disease of the newborn.
D Hodgkin's disease.
E *Mycoplasma pneumoniae* infection.

Question 27 von Willebrand's disease is not characterized by the following:

A Prolonged bleeding time.
B Normal platelet function.
C Recurrent epistaxis.
D Prolonged activated partial thromboplastin time.
E Response to treatment with ddAVP.

Answer 23

E An interstitial pneumonitis.

Myeloma typically causes lytic lesions in the bone. A paraprotein may not be found in up to 20% of people. Renal involvement may include: interstitial nephritis, light chain deposition, amyloidosis, ATN, nephromegaly, and hypercalcaemic deposition. Interstitial pneumonitis can result from drug therapy for myeloma (busulphan). An elevation in ALP should raise the possibility of bony involvement. Plasma cells are the key cells involved in myeloma and are often referred to as 'memory B-cells'. They are characterized by typical 'clock face' nuclei. Plasma cells may not be seen on the bone marrow aspirate and only on trephine biopsy. Malignant change within plasma cells should raise the possibility of plasmacytoma.

Tutorial

See Answer 19.

Answer 24

A Warm haemagglutinin disease.

Infectious mononucleosis is caused by EBV infection. There is splenomegaly with cervical lymphadenopathy and flu-like illness. Red cell agglutination is a common finding and typically occurs at cold temperature. Agglutinins may be misread by the FBC machine and be mistakenly counted as macrocytes, giving a high MCV reading. 'Warm' autoimmune haemolytic antibodies are seen in association with Hodgkin's lymphoma; they result in haemaglutination at room temperature. Abnormal T-lymphocytes are morphologically 'odd' looking on blood film, with an eccentric cytoplasm; they are typically seen in an array of viral infections.

Tutorial

The different ways in which EBV infection manifests clinically should be understood.

Features inlude: B-cell infection, membranous tonsillar exudate, thrombocytopenia and hepatomegaly.

Abnormal T-lymphocytes are seen in: cytomegalovirus infection, infectious mononucleosis, rubella, toxoplasmosis, toxocarosis, and herpes simplex infections.

Answer 25

D Predisposition to infection from encapsulated bacteria.

Sickle cell disease is the homozygous defect of the β-chain of haemoglobin (a substitution of valine for glutamate at position 6). There is usually growth retardation, predisposition to infection by encapsulated bacteria (as the spleen undergoes autoinfarction), and sickle cells in the serum, especially during hypoxic, cold periods. Aplastic crisis is usually precipitated by infection with parvovirus (as this infects early erythrocyte precursors), but rarely may be caused by other viral infections. Proctitis is seen occasionally in adults, whereas dactylitis is more often seen in childhood. Hypo-and not hypersplenism occurs as a result of splenic autoinfarction.

Tutorial

This is a common childhood genetic condition that is often encountered in adult medicine; therefore, the genetic basis and clinical sequelae should be understood.

Features include: dactylitis, short stature, digital amputations (auto), gall stones, chest syndrome. Hydroxyurea may increase the levels of HbF. Crisis may warrant exchange transfusions, otherwise the mainstay of treatment is with folate supplementation and penicillin prophylaxis.

Answer 26

C Haemorrhagic disease of the newborn.

Coombs' test will be positive when antiglobulin is added to blood and a reaction with antibody coated red cells occurs. It usually implies an immune cause of haemolytic anaemia. AIHA is seen in approximately 10% of patients with Hodgkin's disease. *Mycoplasma pneumoniae* can cause a spectrum of extra-respiratory manifestations; these include AIHA, gastrointestinal symptoms, arthralgia, otitis media, and neurological involvement especially affecting the cerebellum. Haemorrhagic disease of the newborn results from a coagulation disorder attributable to vitamin K deficiency.

Tutorial

How the DCT aids in identifying the cause of autoimmune haemolytic anaemia should be understood. Examples include: methyldopa-induced AIHA, transfusion mismatch, rhesus disease of the newborn.

Answer 27

B Normal platelet function.

von Willebrand's disease is an inherited (variable pattern) deficiency of vWF. This factor is a crucial anchoring factor between clotting factors (through factor VIII) and platelets (via IIb/IIIa receptor). Patients usually present to either the ENT surgeon (with recurrent epistaxis) or gynaecologist (with menorrhagia). There is usually a prolonged bleeding time (platelet function) and APTT. There is a transient rise in vWF levels following administration of ddAVP, as stored vWF is released from endothelial cells. Desmopressin is a synthetic analogue of arginine vasopressin, but with fewer pressor effects and a longer half-life *in vivo*.

Tutorial

The relationship between vWF and factor VIII in clot formation from a platelet plug is intricate and should be well understood. Similarity in certain laboratory tests can occur. (See Answer 21.)

Question 28 The following is not associated with spherocytes on the blood film:

A Microangiopathic haemolytic anaemia.
B Sickle cell disease.
C Pyruvate kinase deficiency.
D Glucose-6-phosphate-dehydrogenase deficiency.
E Beta-thalassaemia.

Question 29 The following are true of carcinoid tumours in the GI tract except:

A They are more common in the large bowel.
B Usually cause constipation.
C Inevitably present with flushing and wheezing.
D Are usually localized.
E Metastases are usually to the right lobe of the liver.

Question 30 The following is not true of coeliac disease:

A Can be reliably diagnosed serologically.
B Is associated with an eruptive skin rash.
C Is common in the Celtic population.
D Is associated with Howell–Jolly bodies on the blood film.
E Causes a macrocytic anaemia.

Question 31 The following is least useful in the diagnosis of malabsorption:

A Barium swallow.
B Enteroscopy.
C Pancreo-lauryl test.
D H_2 breath test.
E Height/weight charts.

Answer 28

D Glucose-6-phosphate-dehydrogenase deficiency.

G6PD deficiency is the only haemolytic anaemia not associated with spherocytes on the blood film. Spherocytes are characterized by normocytic hyperchromatic indices. Heinz bodies are the finding in G6PD deficiency.

Tutorial

The presence of spherocytes on a blood film is a normal response to haemolysis.

MAHA features include: anaemia, spherocytes, fragment cells, and thrombocytopenia.

Answer 29

B Usually cause constipation.

Carcinoid tumours are equally common in men and women. They are most frequently found at the tip of the appendix. Although usually solitary, they can be multifocal in up to 40% of cases. The carcinoid syndrome occurs when the tumour metastasizes to the liver. The right lobe generally has a larger feeding tributary of the portal vein and hence receives a greater blood flow. The usual symptoms are flushing and diarrhoea accompanied by wheezing.

Tutorial

Neuroendocrine tumours are rare and consequently extensive knowledge is not required. However, students must understand the metabolic basis of the clinical features, and that they only manifest once liver metastases develop, as the product of these tumours, 5-HIAA, undergoes extensive first-pass metabolism.

Phaeochromocytoma features: raised levels of urinary VMA and nor- and epinephrine.

Answer 30

A Can be reliably diagnosed serologically.

Coeliac disease is more common in the Celtic population and is caused by a sensitivity to gluten in the diet. There are characteristic autoantibody associations (antigliadin and antiendomysial) but definitive diagnosis requires an intraluminal biopsy of the jejunum prior to a gluten-free diet. It is associated with dermatitis herpetiformis which is an exquisitely pruritic rash, hyposplenism, and the development of small bowel lymphoma. The jejunum and proximal ileum are the main sites of iron absorption. Howell–Jolly bodies are seen in sera of patients with hyposplenism; they imply a failure to clear red blood cell breakdown. A macrocytic anaemia is seen due to failure to absorb folate adequately, which mainly occurs in the upper intestine (duodeno-jejuno flexure and proximal jejunum).

Tutorial

Coeliac disease is not a typical autoimmune disorder. The autoantibodies associated with it have not been shown to be pathogenic and exchange transfusion does not result in improvement.

Answer 31

E Height/weight charts.

Growth charts are useful in identifying malabsorption but shed no light as to the cause. Barium swallow is a test of anatomical abnormalities in the oesophagus, and requires a follow-through study or small bowel enema to identify anatomical causes of malabsorption. The H_2 breath test will be useful in bacterial overgrowth syndromes and either the pancreo-lauryl or PABA test will identify pancreatic enzyme deficiencies.

Tutorial

Malabsorption is less frequently due to aberrant anatomy than to a functional problem. In the developing world, nutritional intake remains the main problem. In the Western world the main distinction is between intestinal (mucosal) and extra-intestinal causes.

Examples include: jejunal diverticulosis, blind loop syndrome, short bowel syndrome, celiac, tropical sprue, chronic pancreatitis.

Question 32 The following are not true of an isolated positive titre of anti-HepB sAg except:

A It indicates previous infection with Hepatitis B.
B Is suggestive of recent vaccination.
C Is associated with high infectivity.
D Suggests a chronic carrier state.
E Is indicative of active infection.

Question 33 The following is pathognomic of Whipple's disease:

A Oculomhyrrthmias.
B Large joint arthritis.
C Lymphocytic CSF.
D Constipation.
E Cure following radical GI surgery.

Question 34 The following are recognized extra-intestinal features of inflammatory bowel disease except:

A Episcleritis.
B Rheumatoid-type arthritis.
C HLA B27 positivity.
D Pyoderma gangrenosum.
E Erythema nodosum.

Question 35 The following is true of *H. pylori*:

A It is similar morphologically to *H. influenzae*.
B Affects the immunocompromised.
C Is less common in smokers.
D Protects against the development of duodenal adenocarcinoma.
E Is more commonly problematic in the developing world.

Question 36 The following is not true of Crohn's disease:

A Disease activity can be assessed clinically.
B The CRP is raised even during remission.
C Acute treatment involves steroid enema therapy.
D Is a cause of megacolon on abdominal X-ray.
E Is a greater risk for small bowel cancer than ulcerative colitis.

Answer 32

B Is suggestive of recent vaccination.

The HepB sAg is present in the serum early in the course of disease and usually disappears within 6 months. Its continuing presence for longer than 6 months implies chronic infection. The presence of eAg indicates high infectivity whilst presence of anti-HepB sAg alone implies vaccination. The presence of anti-HepB sAg alone does not indicate previous infection, as it will also be present in the sera of those who have been vaccinated against hepatitis B.

Answer 33

A Oculomhyrrthmias.

Whipple's disease is caused by *Tropheryma whipplei*, and is characterized by the triad of spondyloarthritis, diarrhoea, and neurological sequelae. Writhing movements of the tongue are virtually pathognomic of the disease. Whipple's disease is a cause of lymphocytic CSF.

Tutorial

Whipple's disease is unrelated to the pancreas. The neurological manifestations are multisystem and often occur late. Diagnosis usually requires PCR amplification of DNA in CSF.

Lymphocytic CSF is associated with: viral infections, *Legionella* spp., spirochaetal disease, SLE, demyelinating disease, brucellosis, TB, Hodgkin's lymphoma, Behçet's disease, NSAIDs, and heavy metal poisoning.

Answer 34

B Rheumatoid-type arthritis.

Extra-intestinal manifestations occur in 5–10% of patients with inflammatory bowel disease, and can represent disease activity in some patients. The characteristic eye findings are of anterior uveitis (especially episcleritis). The arthritis is associated with HLAB27 positivity and resembles that of the other seronegative (rheumatoid factor) spondyloarthritides (large weight bearing joints). The skin manifestations include both pyoderma gangrenosum and erythema nodosum.

Tutorial

Crohn's disease affects all layers of the bowel wall, and is associated with more florid disease (fissuring, fistulating disease, abscess formation). Terminal ileum involvement is characteristic. UC affects the mucosa only and gives the characteristic cobblestone mucosa appearance on radiography. Morbidity is usually less in the latter.

Pyoderma gangrenosum is associated with: DM, myeloma, paraproteinaemia, Hodgkin's disease, UC, Crohn's, rheumatoid arthritis, and Wegener's granulomatosis.

Erythema nodosum is associated with: sarcoid, Behçet's, rheumatoid arthritis, TB, leprosy, brucellosis, histoplasmosis, coccidiomycosis, drug reaction (dapsone, sulphonamides), and streptococcal infection.

Answer 35

A It is similar morphologically to *H. influenzae.*

Helicobacter pylori is a cocco-bacillus which morphologically resembles both *H. influenzae* and *Campylobacter jejuni*. It is found in the majority of cases mainly in the Western world in fully immunocompetent people, who may be asymptomatic. Smoking seems to offer little protection against colonization and there seems to be a tentative association with duodenal carcinoma.

Tutorial

H. pylori is an important vibrio bacteria that is highly linked to gastrointestinal disease: atrophic gastritis, ulcerative disease, and carcinoma.

Tests include: serological, urease breath test, biopsy and culture, biopsy and PCR.

Answer 36

B The CRP is raised even during remission.

Tutorial

The aetiology and pathogenesis of inflammatory bowel disease have not been fully elucidated. It is fair to say that Crohn's and UC are two diseases on a spectrum.

Extra-intestinal manifestations in Crohn's disease are often used to determine disease activity clinically. Unlike UC, the CRP is raised during active infection and is absent during disease quiescence. Azathioprine therapy takes 6–12 months to be effective and is not indicated in the acute treatment of the disease, where topical and or systemic steroids or parenteral nutrition are more effective. Megacolon is a radiological sign associated with UC. UC presents no excess risk to the development of small bowel cancer.

Question 37 The following is true of ulcerative colitis but not Crohn's disease:

A High output entero-enteric fistulae are common.
B Biopsy reveals crypt abscess in the submucosa.
C Fissures are more common on barium meals.
D Smokers have fewer relapses than nonsmokers.
E Toxic megacolon is less likely to occur.

Question 38 The following conditions increase the risk of developing malignant bowel cancer except:

A Li–Fraumeni syndrome.
B Familial adenomatous polyposis.
C Gardner's syndrome.
D Peutz–Jegher's syndrome.
E Smoking.

Questions 39–41 A 72-year-old widower was seen in clinic complaining of weight loss, malaise, and recent diarrhoea. He was a previous heavy smoker but suffered with no other medical ailments. However, systems enquiry revealed in addition a recent history of back pain.

Question 39 The following would all be suitable initial investigations to perform except:

A Colonoscopy + biopsy.
B CXR.
C Isotope bone scan.
D Stool cytology.
E Serum electrophoresis.

Question 40 Which of the following would least explain his back pain:

A Osteoporosis.
B Sclerotic metastasis.
C Osteomalacia.
D Hyperparathyroidism.
E Paget's disease.

Question 41 The following are all possible underlying diagnoses except:

A Squamous cell carcinoma of the anus.
B Duke's C adenocarcinoma of the sigmoid colon.
C Metastatic adenocarcinoma of the rectum.
D Adenocarcinoma of the prostate.
E Duke's B adenocarcinoma of the rectum.

Answer 37

D Smokers have fewer relapses than nonsmokers.

Fistulating and fissuring disease is more characteristic of Crohn's disease. Smoking is protective in UC but predisposes to the development of Crohn's. In the absence of characteristic radiographic evidence, a full thickness biopsy will be required. Megacolon is a radiological sign more frequently associated with UC.

Tutorial

See Answers 34 and 36.

Answer 38

D Peutz–Jegher's syndrome.

Li–Fraumeni syndrome is an inherited cancer syndrome caused by loss of the p53 gene (TP53), and hence a vital tumour suppressor gene. Virtually all tumours are more likely. FAP and Gardner's are both inherited forms of large bowel adenocarcinoma. Peutz–Jegher's causes small bowel hamartomas. Smoking increases the risk of developing most cancers.

Other inheritable cancer syndromes include xeroderma pigmentosa, neurofibromatosis I and II, and Wilms' syndrome.

Answer 39

D Stool cytology.

Presentation of weight loss with recently altered bowel habit should alert to the possibility of a left-sided colonic tumour. The investigations initially therefore should include a sigmoidoscopy and/or barium enema (CT enema/virtual colonoscopy is currently on trial). Stool cytology although noninvasive is likely to be negative, as it has a poor yield. A CXR is always appropriate in the investigation of any patient with a suspected underlying malignancy, in order to determine whether metastatic lesions are evident (the lung is a site for spread from a multitude of primary malignancies including bowel). An isotope bone scan will reveal areas of focal and generalized uptake of radiomarkers, and is a reliable way of investigating the cause of bone pain thought to be due to metastatic deposits in bone. Serum electrophoresis will reveal the presence of a paraproteinaemia, which should be in the differential diagnosis of a possible malignancy in this age group.

Answer 40

E Paget's disease.

Hyperparathyroidism usually presents with constipation but diarrhoea may occur from overflow. Paget's disease tends to involve the pelvic girdle before the spine and is not commonly associated with GI upset, with systemic effects usually relating to the heart. Osteoporosis would not be expected to cause diarrhoea or dramatic weight loss. Sclerotic metastases are seen with prostatic carcinoma; diarrhoea would be an unusual way for prostatic carcinoma to present. Osteomalacia typically presents in the Asian population with a painful proximal myopathy.

Answer 41

E Duke's B adenocarcinoma of the rectum.

Duke's B tumours are confined to the bowel wall and therefore could not account for the back pain. All of the other options could explain the back pain. Squamous cell carcinoma of the anus readily metastasizes to the inguinal lymph nodes in 50% of cases, but bony metastases are uncommon.

Tutorial

Duke originally developed his classification for rectal tumours. As the rectum in part strictly speaking has no serosa, the classification has been modified to encompass the remainder of the colon, where there is a serosal covering.

Duke's classification: A: confined to mucosa; B: breach mucosa; C: reach local nodes/ pelvic spread; [D: distant spread – there was no stage D in the original Duke's classification].

Question 42 The following are not true of Wenkebach's phenomenon except:

A Progressive shortening of P-R interval.
B Fixed 2:1 block.
C Tachycardia.
D Extra beat after PR lengthening.
E Is an indication for a temporary pacemaker.

Question 43 The following is the most consistent recognized ECG manifestation of hypocalcaemia:

A Tachycardia.
B Prolonged PR interval.
C Prolonged QT interval.
D Presence of U waves.
E Slurred upstroke to the QRS complex.

Question 44 The following are all clinical features of infective endocarditis except:

A Anaemia.
B Roth spots.
C Hepatosplenomegaly.
D Microscopic haematuria.
E Tricuspid regurgitation.

Question 45 The following is least likely to present with a pericardial rub:

A Acute renal failure.
B Radiation therapy.
C Tuberculosis.
D Rheumatic fever.
E Coxsackie virus A16.

Question 46 The following would be inconsistent with an ECG suggesting acute pulmonary embolus:

A Left ventricular hypertrophy.
B Right bundle branch block.
C Right ventricular hypertrophy.
D Right axis deviation.
E Atrial fibrillation.

Answer 42

E Is an indication for a temporary pacemaker.

Tutorial

This question tests the student's ability to differentiate between the causes of atrio-ventricular conduction block.

Wenkebach phenomenon (Mobitz type I) second degree AV block is characterized by progressive lengthening of the P-R interval, followed by a missed beat and subsequent reduction of the P-R interval in the ensuing captured beat. Unlike Mobitz II second degree AV block (fixed block), the likelihood of degeneration to complete heart block is low and so there is no indication for a permanent pacemaker. Clearly tachycardia is incompatible with pure heart block.

Answer 43

C Prolonged QT interval.

Tutorial

Students should be able to recognize some of the ECG features of hypocalcaemia, hypokalaemia, and hypomagnesaemia.

Clinical features include: tetany, carpopedal spasm, oral paraesthesiae, Chvostek's sign (tapping of facial nerve), Trousseau's sign (inflation of BP cuff precipitates carpopedal spasm).

Hypocalacemia is most consistently associated with prolongation of the QT interval although ST segment abnormalities and U waves are also recognized in severe cases. A prolonged PR interval and U waves are more characteristic features of hypokalaemia. Tachycardia is a nonspecific feature that can occur in many conditions. A slurred upstroke to the QRS complex is a feature of the presence of an accessory pathway between the atria and ventricles, as in the Wolff–Parkinson–White syndrome.

Answer 44

D Microscopic haematuria.

Tutorial

The commonest presentation of endocarditis is that of a septic illness and the finding of a cardiac murmur.

Microscopic haematuria features include: gomerulonephritides, trauma, march haemoglobinuria.

Anaemia (conjunctival pallor), Roth spots (fundoscopy), and hepatosplenomegaly can all be detected clinically. Thrombocytopenia may occur in infective endocarditis especially with large fungal vegetations, as part of MAHA. However, like microscopic haematuria, it is not evident on clinical examination. Tricuspid regurgitation will typically produce a pansystolic murmur and may be associated with systolic waves in the JVP waveform.

Answer 45

A Acute renal failure.

Tutorial

All the responses are causes of a pericardial rub. However, students should recognize that the wider availability of haemofiltration has resulted in uraemia being treated before it becomes severe enough to cause acute pericarditis.

A pericardial rub is heard when there is an inflammatory process within the pericardium. Tuberculosis is the commonest worldwide cause of pericarditis and is not an infrequent finding in recent immigrants and, now in the UK increasingly, the elderly population. Coxsackie virus causes a myocarditis, which usually manifests as a sleeping tachycardia, though a pericarditic process may occur secondarily. Rheumatic fever can cause a pancarditis (Ducket–Jones major criteria). Acute renal failure will cause a pericardial rub only in the presence of uraemia, and these days haemofiltration is commenced prior to its presence.

Answer 46

A Left ventricular hypertrophy.

The commonest ECG finding in PE is sinus tachycardia. Less frequently, right-sided changes (RBBB, RVH, RAD) are seen. Atrial fibrillation is a well recognized presentation of acute PE. LVH may coexist in a patient with an acute PE but an underlying history of hypertension or aortic stenosis should be sought. The CXR finding is commonly normal.

Tutorial

Neither the ECG or chest radiograph are reliable diagnostic tools; often the diagnosis is made on the degree of clinical suspicion.

Tests used: V/Q scan (looking for ventilation/perfusion mismatches), high resolution spiral CT of the chest, spiral CT pulmonary angiogram, or duplex ultrasonography to locate a source of deep vein thrombus.

Question 47 All of the following are indications for a temporary pacing wire with the exception of:

A Recurrent bradycardic episodes with associated collapse.
B Third degree AV block.
C Bradycardia following inferior MI.
D Bifascicular block following large anterior MI.
E Mobitz type II block.

Question 48 The following parameters cannot be obtained directly by placement of a Swann–Ganz catheter:

A Pulmonary artery pressure.
B Mean left atrial pressure.
C Right atrial pressure.
D Systemic vascular resistance.
E Cardiac index.

Question 49 The following is the least recognized feature of mitral stenosis:

A Cough.
B Hoarse voice.
C Dysphagia.
D Haemoptysis.
E Third heart sound.

Question 50 The following is least likely to be attributed to digoxin therapy:

A Nausea.
B Gynaecomastia.
C Galactorrhoea.
D Impotence.
E Red/green colour blindness.

Answer 47

C Bradycardia following inferior MI.

Patients with recurrent syncope associated with synchronous arrhythmia are likely to benefit most from a pacemaker. Following an acute inferior MI (affecting predominantly the right ventricle), bradycardia is a frequent finding. However, this is usually responsive to treatment with atropine and does not require pacing.

Tutorial

Indications for PPM include: Mobitz II block, bifascicular block after anterior MI, complete heart block, sick sinus syndrome.

Most people would, however, place a temporary pacing wire if the bradycardia did not resolve within 2 weeks.

Answer 48

B Mean left atrial pressure.

A Swann–Ganz catheter is indicated when knowledge of the function of the left ventricle is desirable (i.e. when it is felt that the function of the right ventricle cannot be used as a surrogate marker). The mean LAP cannot be obtained but the pulmonary artery capillary wedge pressure can be used as a surrogate instead. The catheter has at least three probes (RA pressure, temperature probe, wedge pressure probe). From these data the cardiac output can be calculated (Fick principle) and also the systemic vascular resistance (the blood pressure can be measured or more frequently is obtained directly from an arterial line reading). The cardiac index is the cardiac output/m^2.

Tutorial

The question tests an understanding of invasive monitoring in relation to cardiovascular physiology. Students should be able to know with confidence when such invasive monitoring might be indicated, and the parameters that can be modified on a real-time basis.

Indications include ARDS, when blood pressure is seemingly unresponsive to simple inotropes, and when adequate venous filling fails to maintain a mean arterial pressure (i.e. when Starling's law is not being followed as expected).

Answer 49

E Third heart sound.

The enlarged left atrium may compress the left main bronchus causing cough and haemoptysis. Compression of the recurrent laryngeal nerve as it passes under the left main bronchus may cause a hoarse voice. Compression of the oesophagus may cause dysphagia.

Tutorial

Students are being tested to see if they recognize that the presence of S_3 in association with mitral stenosis signifies an additional component.

S_3 may be present in the following: mitral regurgitation, LVF, and a young fit healthy person (normal).

Answer 50

E Red/green colour blindness.

Nausea and vomiting are the commonest side-effects of digoxin. Impotence and gynaecomastia occur as a result of high oestrogen levels. Yellow-green achromoptopsia occurs. Red-green is lost early in optic neuritis. Galactorrhoea is milky discharge from the nipple and, like impotence, is attributed to the antioestrogen effect of digoxin.

ECG features of digoxin therapy include: 'reverse tick' in lateral chest leads, ST depression, short P-R interval, ventricular bigemini/trigemini, and nodal bradycardia (toxicity).

Question 51 The following is not a common feature of hypertensive retinopathy:

A Flame shaped haemorrhage.
B Arterio-venous nipping.
C Vitreous haemorrhage.
D Papilloedema.
E Silver wiring.

Question 52 The following are true of proteinuria except:

A >50 g/l is required for the diagnosis of nephritic syndrome.
B Microalbuminuria is the earliest detectable finding in type 2 diabetic nephropathy.
C Causes an early morning frothy urine.
D In the young healthy female, orthostatic hypotension may be a cause.
E Does not always indicate underlying kidney disease.

Question 53 In the diuretic phase of acute tubular necrosis the following are true except:

A Urine is dilute and alkaline.
B There is naturesis.
C Urine contains casts.
D Tamm–Horsfall protein is likely to be present.
E Renal dose dopamine is contraindicated.

Question 54 The following is not characteristic of the nephrotic syndrome:

A A procoagulant state.
B Low levels of LDL and VLDL cholesterol.
C Periorbital oedema is common.
D Serum albumin is <30 g/l.
E The commonest cause in a young boy is likely to be minimal change glomerulonephritis.

Question 55 The following may be causal factors in metabolic alkalosis except:

A Hyperkalaemia.
B Prolonged vomiting.
C Ulcerative colitis.
D Mineralocorticoid excess.
E Villous adenoma of the colon.

Answer 51

C Vitreous haemorrhage.

Hypertensive retinopathy is classified as follows:
- Grade I – Increased vessel tortuosity.
- Grade II – A–V nipping, flame shaped haemorrhages.
- Grade III – Silver wiring.
- Grade IV – Papilloedema.

Diabetic retinopathy features include a background of dot and blot haemorrhages, and cotton-wool spots.

Preproliferative features include neovascularization; proliferative features include florid haemorrhages. Maculopathy is present when the above changes are visualized in the area of the fovea.

Answer 52

A >50 g/l is required for the diagnosis of nephritic syndrome.

Nephritic syndrome usually heralds underlying glomerular pathology. It consists of hypertension and microscopic haematuria. There may in addition be proteinuria, but levels >35 g/l are usually more characteristic of nephrotic syndrome. Microalbuminuria is the earliest biochemical finding in diabetic nephropathy, and is seen in both type 1 and 2. An early morning frothy urine is highly suggestive of proteinuria. In the young fit adolescent, protein in the urine may be posturally related. This benign condition should only be diagnosed when there is a detectable difference in postural urinary collections.

Tutorial

Students should be able to define proteinuria, and recognize that in most but not all circumstances, it represents a pathological finding.

Answer 53

A Urine is dilute and alkaline.

Acute tubular necrosis consists of an initial oliguric phase, where the urine is concentrated and of small volume, with low urinary sodium, and a diuretic phase where urine volumes are large and dilute. The urinary pH is low and there is naturesis. The urine may contain tubular casts and Tamm–Horsfall protein. Dopamine in low-medium dose (2–5 μg/kg) will increase renal perfusion and is used (by some) in the oliguric phase to increase urine production.

Tutorial

The ability to identify the different phases of acute tubular necrosis is being tested here, with the associated differing biochemical profiles in the blood and urine.

Answer 54

B Low levels of LDL and VLDL cholesterol.

The nephrotic syndrome is characterized by hypoalbuminuria (<30 g/l), proteinuria (>35 g/l), and oedema. There is in addition, hypercholesterolaemia. The cause in the young is usually minimal change GN, and in the adult membranous GN. The loss of protein is accompanied by loss of larger proteins, in particular antithrombin III, resulting in a prothrombotic state.

Tutorial

Students should be able to define the proteinuria threshold for the diagnosis of the nephrotic syndrome and the serious indirect sequelae that result.

Causes of nephrotic syndrome include: membranoproliferative GN, SLE, DM, drugs (gold, penicillamine), focal segmental GN.

Answer 55

A Hyperkalaemia.

The crucial role of the tubular system of the nephron is to conserve sodium. Most Na^+ is reabsorbed in the proximal tubule; that which is not is reabsorbed in exchange for both H^+ and K^+ ions in the distal tubule. In addition, the aldosterone effect to exchange Na^+ for K^+ occurs in the proximal collecting tubules. In vomiting and diarrhoea (e.g. with UC, villous adenoma of colon), the loss of H^+ is accompanied by loss of Na^+ which triggers the kidney to conserve more, resulting in hypokalaemia, and a paradoxical aciduria. The physiological exchange across membranes between H^+ and K^+ has a net effect of causing a metabolic acidosis in hyperkalaemia. The single most useful test in hypokalaemic metabolic alkalosis is a urinary K^+ level, as this will help identify the origin of loss (bowel versus kidney). Mineralocorticoid excess results in excess secretion of K^+ and H^+ in the distal tubule, by an agonist effect at the aldosterone receptor or intracellular second messenger systems.

Tutorial

The kidney's primary objective is to conserve sodium and by doing so it preserves the extracellular osmolarity and volume. Consequently, a major control mechanism exists in the distal tubule in the form of the aldosterone mediated $Na^+/K^+/H^+$ ion pump.

Question 56 Rapidly proliferative glomerulonephritis may occur as a consequence of all the following except:

A Infective endocarditis.
B Malignant hypertension.
C Recent streptococcal infection.
D Cryoglobulinaemia.
E Henoch–Schönlein purpura.

Question 57 Nephromegaly is least likely to be seen in:

A Myeloma.
B Type 2 NIDDM.
C Non-Hodgkin's lymphoma.
D Sickle cell disease.
E Acromegaly.

Question 58 The following is not true of renal cell carcinoma:

A Anaemia may be present.
B Polycythaemia may be present.
C Pel–Ebstein fever is rarely seen.
D Spindle cell variety has a favourable prognosis.
E Large solitary metastases may be found in the lung.

Question 59 The following are recognized causes of magnesium depletion except:

A Therapy with carboplatin.
B Prolonged parenteral feeding.
C Diabetic ketoacidosis.
D Ulcerative colitis.
E Hypokalaemia.

Question 60 The following are not recognized characteristics of kidney involvement in multiple myeloma except:

A A positive nitrogen balance.
B Usually associated hypertension.
C Interstitial nephritis may occur as a result of hypercalcaemia.
D Reversible by treating the myeloma.
E Haematuria is more common than proteinuria.

Answer 56

E Henoch–Schönlein purpura.

RPGN is associated with crescent formation within the glomerulus, and is a cause of rapid renal decline. It may follow 2–3 weeks after streptococcal infection, as an immune complex disease, or be consequent to grade IV hypertension. Immune complex formation in infective endocarditis and cryoglobulinaemia accounts for the renal involvement in these conditions. HSP is associated with IgA deposition and not crescentric RPGN.

Tutorial

The common causes of RPGN should be known, as should the presentation with the nephritic syndrome (hypertension, haematuria, red cell casts in the urine). SLE commonly affects the kidney (lupus nephritis) but usually causes a more subacute nephritis that may go on to decline rapidly, but is not usually associated with crescent formation.

Answer 57

D Sickle cell disease.

Lupus nephritis causes a reduction in renal mass, as does HbSS (autoinfarction). In acromegly there is generalized organomegaly. Myeloma and NIDDM can both cause nephromegaly. Other causes include hydronephrosis, renal vein thrombosis, and lymphoma.

Tutorial

Nephromegaly can be attributable to increased functioning or organ infiltration. Renal artery stenosis will lead to small atrophied kidneys.

Answer 58

D Spindle cell variety has a favourable prognosis.

Renal adenocarcinoma usually occurs during the 5th–6th decade. The classical triad of haematuria, loin pain, and a mass is seen in <30% of people. Both anaemia and polycythaemia may occur, the latter as a consequence of erythropoietin production in the tumour. The Pel–Ebstein fever may also be seen (sustained daily fevers, followed by a week of quiescence and then fevers again). The spindle cell type on histology has the least favourable prognosis Cannonball metastases in the lung may respond to treatment of the primary tumour.

Tutorial

The Pel–Ebstein fever is also seen in TB and Hodgkin's disease.

Answer 59

E Hypokalaemia.

Magnesium levels generally mirror those of potassium, whilst the effect of magnesium tends to reflect that of calcium. However, hypokalaemia per se does not cause hypomagnesaemia. Carboplatin (used in chemotherapy for ovarian carcinoma) has toxic effects on the distal tubule where magnesium transport is coordinated. In UC, magnesium is lost in diarrhoea to a level equal to and sometimes greater than potassium. Prolonged parenteral nutrition results in a deficiency of both magnesium and phosphate ions, as does diabetic ketoacidosis.

Clinical features include: paraesthesia, ventricular arrhythmia, muscle spasm.

Answer 60

C Interstitial nephritis may occur as a result of hypercalcaemia.

Myeloma may affect the kidney in a number of ways: interstitial nephritis from deposition of calcium, β_2-microglobin, or light chains; glomerulonephritis; amyloidosis; antimyeloma chemotherapy agents; or by increased susceptibility to infection. There is a negative nitrogen balance, and hypertension is unusual. The kidney disease does not improve in line with the haematological disease when treated with either chemotherapy or bone marrow transplant. The nephrotic syndrome is more likely than the nephritic and hence proteinuria often accompanies the kidney disease.

Treatment of myeloma is usually with an alkylating agent (melphalan/busulphan) or allograft bone marrow transplantation. Treatment of myeloma kidney is usually with CAPD.

Question 61 The following statement is true of digoxin:

A The commonest side-effect is yellow/green xanthopsia.
B The presence of a 'reverse tick' on the ECG signifies digoxin toxicity.
C Ventricular bigemini is often seen on the ECG.
D When used in the treatment of fast atrial fibrillation, produces chemical cardioversion.
E Only indicated in patients with atrial fibrillation and normal cardiac function.

Question 62 The drug least likely to act as an enzyme inducer is:

A Phenytoin.
B Rifampicin.
C Carbamazepine.
D Phenobarbitone.
E Warfarin.

Question 63 The following statement is true:

A A higher dose of azathioprine is required when given to patients being treated for gout.
B A higher dose of warfarin will be required in patients taking erythromycin.
C Warfarin reduces the action of aspirin.
D Carbamazepine will induce its own metabolism.
E Trimethoprim interferes with folate absorption.

Question 64 Features of phenytoin toxicity include all of the following except:

A Hirsutism.
B Truncal ataxia.
C Limb dysmetria.
D Supraventricular tachycardia.
E Seizures.

Answer 61

C Ventricular bigemini is often seen on the ECG.

Digoxin is a cardiac glycoside, derived from the Foxglove plant product, digitalis. It has a number of functions, namely to act as a positive inotrope and a negative chronotrope. It does the latter by primarily delaying AV nodal conduction, though it has effects in other parts of the cardiac action potential as well. The primary indication is for rapid atrial fibrillation/flutter, where it gives rate control and does not act to produce chemical cardioversion. The commonest side-effects are of nausea and vomiting with xanthopsia being less frequent. The 'reverse tick' sign is seen with levels of digoxin within the normal therapeutic range. The results of the Digoxin Investigation Group (DIG) trial indicate that digoxin was most effective when given to patients with coexisting heart failure.

Tutorial

Students are being tested on their clinical understanding of digoxin therapy, its indications and features of toxicity. This should present no difficulty for those with sufficient clinical experience.

Answer 62

E Warfarin.

Warfarin has no effect on the cytochrome oxidase system in the liver. Acute ethanol poisoning may result in ethanol acting as an inducer, the opposite is true in chronic abuse. CBZ induces its own metabolism as well as that of other drugs. Special caution is required when given with other antiepileptic drugs and the COCP.

Tutorial

Some of the clinically important drug interactions should be known, especially those drugs that act in a way to alter the bioavailability of other important drugs (inducers and inhibitors of the hepatic cytochrome p_{450} system of drug metabolism).

- Enzyme inducers: rifampicin, phenytoin, CBZ, valproate.
- Enzyme inhibitors: ciprofloxacin, alcohol, erythromycin.

Answer 63

D Carbamazepine will induce its own metabolism.

A reduced dose of azathioprine is required when given to patients taking allopurinol, as the latter inhibits metabolism of azathioprine and causes high levels of the active metabolite mercaptopurine.

Erythromycin acting as an enzyme inhibitor causes an elevation in the INR, and therefore warfarin dosage should be reduced. Warfarin displaces aspirin from the albumin binding sites. Trimethoprim inhibits dihydrofolate reductase and does not impede folate absorption (unlike phenytoin).

Tutorial

See Answer 62.

Answer 64

A Hirsutism.

Hirsutism, coarse oily skin, acne, gingival hypertrophy, macrocytosis, and osteomalacia are all side-effects of therapy. The development of arrhythmia or neurological signs is suggestive of toxicity, especially truncal ataxia (more specific to phenytoin toxicity than alcohol related cerebellar syndrome).

Tutorial

Students should be able to distinguish between the common sequelae of phenytoin therapy and the features of toxicity.

Truncal ataxia can be easily tested for by asking the patient to sit up from a lying position.

Question 65 The following is not true of warfarin:

A Requires 2–3 days to take effect.
B Toxicity is readily reversed by vitamin K.
C Is metabolized by the liver.
D Is contraindicated in severe hypertension.
E Should be used cautiously in the elderly, as they have increased propensity to develop related complications.

Question 66 The following is true of aspirin:

A Safely causes a reduction in the likelihood of stroke when given as primary prophylaxis.
B Is contraindicated in patients with gastritis.
C Acts by reversibly inhibiting cyclooxygenase.
D Effects are countered by an increase in thromboxane A_2 production.
E Is an aromatic acid derivative.

Question 67 The following are not true of the oxygen dissociation curve except:

A Hypercarbia shifts the curve to the left.
B The Haldane effect describes the effect of O_2 binding in CO poisoning.
C 2,3-DPG shifts the curve to the right.
D A high pH favours tissue oxygenation.
E Chronic hypoxia due to altitude sickness shifts the curve to the left.

Question 68 The following condition increases the transfer factor:

A Asthma.
B Goodpasture's syndrome.
C Chronic bronchitis.
D Smoking.
E Anaemia.

Question 69 The following statement regarding pulmonary manifestations of AIDS is true:

A The commonest infection is with MAI.
B Histoplasmosis pneumonia is common in the south-western USA.
C Allergic bronchopulmonary aspergillosis is more common than systemic aspergillosis.
D Kaposi's sarcoma affects the lung parenchyma.
E Bihilar lymphadenopathy is likely to be due to sarcoidosis.

Answer 65

B Toxicity is readily reversed by vitamin K.

Warfarin irreversibly inhibits clotting factors II, VII, IX, X, as well as proteins S and C. The initial effect is as a procoagulant because of preferential inhibition of the natural anticoagulants, proteins S and C. Effects are reversed readily by fresh frozen plasma and not Vitamin K, which takes 2–3 days to work, as it competitively displaces warfarin from the γ-binding site. Caution is required when prescribing to the elderly, not because of increased sensitivity, but because there is an increased risk of falls in this group, with the concomitant risk of intracranial bleeding. It is contraindicated in liver disease and severe uncontrolled hypertension.

Tutorial

Students should appreciate the key differences in anticoagulation with warfarin and heparin.

Heparin is short acting, reversibly catalyses the action of antithrombin III, and causes alteration in APTT (not LMWH).

Answer 66

B Is contraindicated in patients with gastritis.

Aspirin (acetylsalicylic acid) acts by irreversibly inhibiting cyclooxygenase (COX-1 and COX-2, predominantly gastric). There is a reduction in both prostacyclin and thromboxane A_2 levels. Contraindications include aspirin sensitivity and peptic ulcer disease. Although effective in primary prevention for cerebrovascular disease, the morbidity and risk of gastric complications has resulted in it not being advocated in primary prophylaxis. It is an aromatic acid derivative.

Tutorial

Aspirin is probably the most used drug in medicine and has a therapeutic role in the management of a number of different diseases. Consequently, a comprehensive understanding of how aspirin works and its toxicity in certain situations is necessary. The interaction with warfarin should be understood.

Answer 67

C 2,3-DPG shifts the curve to the right.

Low pH, high lactate, high 2,3-DPG, hypoxia, and hypercarbia all shift the curve to the right. High temperature shifts the curve to the right. The Haldane effect describes the effect of CO_2 on the Hb molecule and its associated solubility.

Tutorial

The student is being asked to demonstrate an understanding of the basic respiratory compensations to varying metabolic circumstances.

The Haldane effect is the enhanced CO_2 diffusibility at low oxygen tensions.

Answer 68

B Goodpasture's syndrome.

Asthma can cause a raised KCO but does not increase the TF. Recent pulmonary haemorrhage in Goodpasture's can raise the TF. Emphysema reduces the TF but pure bronchitis has little effect. Polycythaemia will raise the factor. V/Q mismatches, reducing pulmonary capillary perfusion, will reduce the TF, whereas L-R shunts will have the reverse effect.

Tutorial

Students should understand how the interpretation of the transfer coefficient (TF corrected for lung volume) and other respiratory function tests aid in the diagnosis of respiratory disease. Transfer factor is affected by V/Q mismatch, nature of the alveolar membrane, blood flow in the pulmonary arterial bed, and Hb concentration. Consequently, conditions that result in polycythaemia and pulmonary haemorrhage will result in a raised TF, and anaemia and AV malformations in the lung (such as hereditary haemorrhagic telangiectasia) will result in a reduced TF.

Answer 69

B Histoplasmosis pneumonia is common in the south-western USA.

The commonest lung manifestation in patients with HIV infection is PCP pneumonia, followed by MAI and then TB. Systemic aspergillosis is more common in the AIDS population than ABPA, which is usually associated with an underlying allergic syndrome. Kaposi's sarcoma tends to affect the bronchial vessels rather than the parenchyma. Histoplasmosis is prevalent in cavernous regions where populations of bats may live, such as the desert regions of the USA. In the context of AIDS or when HIV infection is suspected, the presence of bihilar lymphadenopathy should not be attributed to sarcoid without transbronchial biopsy.

Tutorial

AIDS is an important clinical syndrome and the multiorgan sequelae that result from HIV infection should be known. Patients are at risk of developing AIDS when the CD4 count drops to $\leq 200/mm^3$ ($2 \times 10^8/l$). At this stage it is prudent to instigate prophylaxis therapy with septrin.

Question 70 The following statement is correct:

A The carina lies at the level of the 6th thoracic vertebra.
B The carina is fixed with no movement during normal respiration.
C A fixed and raised ipsilateral hemidiaphragm indicates a malignant tumour.
D Surfactant is produced by type II alveolar cells.
E In ARDS the total lung compliance is reduced.

Question 71 The following is true of the measles virus:

A There is an increased risk of autism in people immunized with the measles vaccine.
B There are characteristic intra-oral lesions specific to measles.
C Causes bilateral parotid enlargement.
D Is a DNA virus.
E Has no long term sequelae.

Question 72 The following are causes of pulmonary cavitation except:

A Primary tuberculosis.
B Aspergilloma.
C Small cell lung cancer.
D Infection with *Klebsiella* sp.
E Churg–Strauss disease.

Question 73 The following is true of infection with *Clostridium tetani*:

A Can cause opisthotonus.
B Infects the sensory nerve endings.
C Is a nonsporing Gram-negative bacillus.
D Is now resistant to benzylpenicillin.
E Is an aerobic bacillus that is usually found in soil.

Answer 70

D Surfactant is produced by type II alveolar cells.

The carina lies at the level of the bottom of the 4th thoracic vertebra. It moves with normal inspiration. A fixed ipsilateral hemidiaphragm results from phrenic nerve lesion, which may be due to tumour, a high cervical lesion, or other causes of lymphadenopathy. In ARDS the lung is stiffened and less compliant. Surfactant is produced by type II alveolar cells and improves lung compliance.

Tutorial

A basic knowledge of the main conducting airways is required. The left recurrent laryngeal nerve hooks around the left main bronchus before running cranially, and as such may become infiltrated by tumour. A hoarse voice present for ≥6 weeks should prompt urgent investigation.

Answer 71

B There are characteristic intra-oral lesions specific to measles.

Measles is an RNA virus which typically affects the young population. The prodromal illness is followed by the development of intraoral buccal white lesions (Koplik's spots). Other systemic effect of measles virus include meningitis, arthritis, and encephalitis. Many years after the initial infection there may be an encephalitis syndrome which is immunologically mediated. Despite recent controversy there is no consistent proven link between the MMR vaccine and autism. Unilateral or bilateral parotid enlargement is usually seen in mumps infection.

Tutorial

There are a number of infectious diseases that overlap between childhood and adulthood, and as such may appear in the adult exam. The subacute sclerosing encephalitis that is seen 5–20 years after initial infection with measles virus tends to present with behavioural disturbance or seizures. It can be diagnosed reasonably well on MRI examination.

Other viruses that infect in the child but present in the adult are: mumps, polio, rubella, and Coxsackie.

Answer 72

A Primary tuberculosis.

Lung cavitation in TB occurs in the apices, in areas of previous fibrosis. Infections are the commonest cause of lung cavitation, mostly due to *Staphylococcus aureus* and *Klebsiella* spp. (especially in the immunocompromised patient). Other causes include the systemic vasculitides, tumours, and deep fungal infections.

Tutorial

Primary infection with *Mycobacterium tuberculosis* begin in the lung periphery as a Ghon focus, later forming the Ghon complex when mediastinal lymphadenopathy is present. Reactivation due to immunocompromise results in secondary TB, when lung cavitation is seen.

Answer 73

A Can cause opisthotonus.

Clostridium tetani is a facultative anaerobe found in soil. Once inoculation occurs, the bacterium travels through motor nerve endings and causes damage by infecting the inhibitory interneurones in the spinal cord. Treatment is with wound toileting, and intravenous benzylpenicillin. Human Ig may be beneficial but data is inconsistent. Opisthotonous is a decerebrate posture and is lethal. The 'risus sardonicus' facies are more commonly seen in patients in the Far East.

Tutorial

The student is required to distinguish the clinical syndromes attributable to the different clostridia species.

C. botulinum: NMJ blockade; *C. tetani*: CNS inhibitor of the inhibitory interneurones; C. *welchii* and *C. perfringens*: wound infection, subcutaneous emphysema; *C. difficile*: pseudomembranous colitis.

Question 74 The following is not true of botulinum toxin:

A Toxin has a therapeutic role in Huntington's disease.
B It causes neuromuscular blockade.
C Is a form of food poisoning.
D Can be treated with intravenous high dose penicillin.
E Can be effectively prevented by immunization.

Question 75 The following statement regarding meningitis is true:

A The commonest pathogens in the neonatal period are the group A streptococci.
B In the childhood period, *H. influenzae* is the commonest pathogen.
C The 'meningovax' meningococcal vaccine prevents meningococcal meningitis.
D *N. meningitidis* is a Gram-positive coccus.
E The presence of a petechial rash is diagnostic of meningococcal septicaemia.

Question 76 The following viruses have been implicated in the aetiology of the cancers listed with the exception of:

A EBV and Burkitt's lymphoma.
B CMV and bowel cancer.
C HTLV-I and T-cell leukaemia/lymphoma.
D Herpes virus and Kaposi's sarcoma.
E Hepatitis C virus and hepatocellular carcinoma.

Question 77 The following condition does not cause an elevated αFP:

A Ovarian fibroma.
B Testicular teratoma.
C Hydatidiform mole.
D Squamous cell carcinoma of the lung.
E Liver cirrhosis.

Question 78 The following are recognized risk factors for the subsequent development of oesophageal cancer with the exception of:

A Hyperkeratotic soles of the feet.
B Iron deficiency anaemia.
C Smoking.
D Barrett's oesophagus.
E Middle Eastern origin.

Answer 74

E Can be effectively prevented by immunization.

Botulism is caused by infection with *Clostridium* spp.. It is usually a form of food poisoning, acquired from canned meats. It acts by blocking transmission at the neuromuscular junction and hence causes a flaccid weakness. Treatment is as for other clostridial infections (high-dose penicillin).

Tutorial

The exotoxin of this clostridia has found medicinal usage for the treatment of spasticity associated with dystonic disorders. Commercially it is requested for usage in certain plastic surgery procedures (Botox).

Answer 75

B In the childhood period, *H. influenzae* is the commonest pathogen.

Meningitis in the neonatal period is more likely to be due to group B streptococci (commensals of the birth canal). During childhood *H. influenzae* is a commoner cause. Meningococcus is however, common throughout all ages but affects the adolescent population and elderly more. The meningococcus (*N. meningitidis*) is a Gram-negative coccus. Petechial rashes are seen in septicaemia from other species as well and is not diagnostic of meningococcemia. The meningovax vaccine is effective in preventing meningitis from only certain subtypes of the meningococcus.

Tutorial

Different bacteria are implicated in meningitis at different times of life. The most common *Neiserria* spp. is a group B meningococcus, for which no vaccine is currently available. If the diagnosis of meningitis is clinically suspected, then immediate antibiotic therapy should be instituted.

Answer 76

B CMV and bowel cancer.

EBV has been linked with Burkitt's lymphoma. HTLV-1 is prevalent in Japan (where it tends to cause CNS problems) and Jamaica (where leukaemia is commoner). Recently, HHSV-8 DNA has been identified by PCR from Kaposi's lesions. Hepatitis C causes chronic liver disease and hepatocellular carcinoma especially in south east Asia.

Tutorial

Oncogenes were first identified as being mutated forms of genes normally present (proto-oncogenes) from the work of Peyton Rous. Initially it was thought that viruses carried these genes and inserted them into the host DNA. Oncogenes resulted from activating mutations of proto-oncogenes whereas tumour suppressor genes were identified by inactivating mutations, thus requiring both copies of the proto-oncogene to be mutated.

Oncogenes include: *ras*, *fap*; tumour suppressor genes include: TP53, RB (retinoblastoma gene).

Answer 77

A Ovarian fibroma.

α-FP is a nonspecific marker of HCC, as it is raised to moderate levels in chronic liver disease, lung cancer, COPD, and is also used as a marker for testicular teratoma. β-HCG is a marker for certain rare forms of testicular seminoma and hydatidiform mole.

Tutorial

Tumour markers include: Ca 19-9 (ovarian), CEA (colonic metastases), PSA (prostate), 5-HIAA (carcinoid), VMA (phaeochromocytoma).

Answer 78

B Iron deficiency anaemia.

Tylosis is a hereditary condition causing hyperkeratosis of the palms and soles of feet and has been found to be strongly associated with oesophageal cancer. The Plummer–Vinson syndrome is the association of oesophageal webs and iron deficiency anaemia. Iron deficiency anaemia itself does not confer a greater risk. Barrett's oesophagus is the metaplasia seen in the distal oesophagus as a result of chronic acid insult to the columnar epithelium, that is seen in approximately 30% of cases of reflux oesophagitis. Smoking is implicated in the development of both metaplasia and oesophageal cancer. There is a belt spanning across the middle of the globe, to include the Middle East, where the disease is commonest.

Tutorial

The prevalence of oesophageal cancer is seemingly increasing and as the prognosis is very poor, it is important to recognize the premalignant associations of this tumour. There is an approximately 40% increased risk of oesophageal cancer in patients with Barrett's oesophagus.

Question 79 The following are causes of a mass in the anterior mediastinum with the exception of:

A Teratoma.
B Thymoma.
C Metastatic large cell carcinoma of the lung.
D Neurofibroma.
E Parathyroid adenoma.

Question 80 Marfan's syndrome involves all of the following except:

A Retinal abnormalities of the eye.
B Progressive heart failure.
C Abnormality in the extracellular matrix.
D Scoliosis.
E Venous thrombotic tendency.

Question 81 Features of juvenile RA include all the following except:

A Swinging fevers.
B Lymphadenopathy.
C Pleuritic chest pain.
D Seropositivity for rheumatoid factor.
E Splenomegaly.

Question 82 The following statement regarding osteoarthritis is true:

A Grade III changes imply joint space narrowing.
B Grade II changes are consistent with osteophyte formation.
C There is no familial tendency.
D Hip replacement for osteoarthritis of the hip is beneficial in only 50% of people.
E Commonly affects males more than females.

Question 83 These ophthalmologic findings are all features of SLE except:

A Macular degeneration.
B Scleritis.
C Scleromalacia perforans.
D Seafan retinopathy.
E Optic atrophy.

Answer 79

D Neurofibroma.

The mediastinum is the space between the root of the neck to the top of the diaphragm, in the space created between the lung roots. It is divided into superior and inferior by a line drawn from the lower border of the 4th thoracic vertebra. The inferior mediastinum is further divided into anterior, medial, and posterior, based on relations to the pericardium (which makes up the medial compartment). So by definition the lung does not lie within the mediastinum. An ectopic parathyroid may lie in the anterior mediastinum, as do midline teratomas and thymomas. Parahilar lymph node involvement in metastatic bowel cancer would also account for a mass in the anterior mediastinum. Neurofibromas occur on spinal roots, which lie within the posterior mediastinum.

Posterior mediastinal masses may include: aortic aneurysm, lymph node, phaeochromocytoma (10% are extra-adrenal), and vertebral abscess.

Answer 80

E Venous thrombotic tendency.

Marfan's syndrome may be difficult to distinguish from homocystinuria. In the latter the lens dislocation is usually downwards, there is a low IQ, osteoporosis, and a tendency for both venous and arterial thrombosis. Homocystinuria is due to deficiency of cystathione reductase and may be diagnosed by the nitroprusside test, or by measuring serum folate/cystathione levels. There is a defect in fibrillin synthesis (an extracellular matrix component) in Marfan's.

Features of Marfan's include: upward lens dislocation, retinal detachment, tall stature, wing span >height, arachnodactyly, pectus excavatum, scoliosis, aortic root dilatation (causing aortic regurgitation and chronic heart failure) and dissection, and mitral valve prolapse.

Answer 81

D Seropositivity for rheumatoid factor.

Patients suffering with juvenile RA are usually rheumatoid factor-negative. Joint manifestation may otherwise be similar to RA, with the added systemic features of lymphadenopathy, fever, and skin rash, making it difficult to distinguish from a viral prodromal illness. Pleurisy and splenomegaly both feature in the clinical picture in juvenile RA.

Answer 82

B Grade II changes are consistent with osteophyte formation.

Osteoarthritis is probably a multifactorial disease. However, there are certain groups that are more at risk: those with a family history of early onset knee arthritis, the overweight group, and females.

Tutorial

An arbitrary grading system exists for OA:

- Grade I – Subchondral sclerosis.
- Grade II – Osteophyte formation.
- Grade III – Subchondral cyst formation.
- Grade IV – Asymmetrical loss of joint space.

Hip replacement is of great benefit to >95% of patients with OA.

Answer 83

C Scleromalacia perforans.

Macular degeneration may occur as a result of vasculitic ischaemia directly attributable to the disease process, or due to toxicity with hydroxychloroquine. Anterior uveitis (scleritis, episcleritis) is a feature of the seronegative spondyloarthritides. Scleromalacia perforans is seen in rheumatoid arthritis. SLE is one of few cause of a seafan retinopathy (others include sickle cell disease, leukaemia). Optic atrophy is a rare and theoretical complication (anterior ischaemic optic neuropathy from vasculitis).

Tutorial

The student should be able to distinguish between the major multisystem arthopathies based on ophthalmologic findings. SLE is nine times more likely to afflict females, and usually presents with a photosensitive rash. It is not unusual for the first presentation to be with lupus nephritis. The skin and kidney are relatively spared in rheumatoid arthritis. Generally, the only organ for SLE to spare is the liver.

Question 84 The following is not true of the spondyloarthritides:

A Rheumatoid factor is positive.
B The weight-bearing joints are typically involved.
C Anterior uveitis is a common finding.
D An early diastolic murmur may be audible.
E Chest findings may be mistaken for healed tuberculosis.

Question 85 The following statement regarding the thoracic manifestations of RA is not true:

A Pleural fibrosis is the commonest pathology.
B BOOP is a recognized finding.
C Lung cavitation may occur.
D There may be a diffuse pneumonitis.
E Interstitial fibrosis from RA and that occuring secondary to methotrexate therapy are indistinguishable radiographically.

Question 86 The following regarding Wegener's granulomatosis is true:

A Histology often shows caseating granuloma.
B p-ANCA is positive in >90% of patients.
C Lung cavitation is uncommon.
D Patients may suffer from hypoglossal nerve palsy.
E Deafness is unlikely to be of the conductive type.

Question 87 The following is true of a 'normal distribution':

A The mean is the commonest observation.
B 66% of observations lie within 2 SD from the mean.
C The variance is the square root of the mean.
D All the observations within the distribution are normal.
E The standard error of the mean is generally more accurate than the mean.

Answer 84

A Rheumatoid factor is positive.

In all the spondyloarthritides rheumatoid factor is negative. The spondyloarthritides have in common other features: anterior uveitis, apical lung fibrosis, aortic regurgitation, amyloid changes, plantar fasciitis, calcaneal spurs.

Tutorial

The spondyloarthritides are associated with HLA B27 positivity and all have involvement of the weight bearing joints, especially the sacroiliac joints.

Answer 85

A Pleural fibrosis is the commonest pathology.

The commonest lung manifestation in RA is of an exudative pleural effusion. BOOP is a radiological description of end organ damage in the lung seen with an array of clinical conditions such as RA, chemotherapy, and systemic vasculitides. Diffuse pneumonitis may present clinically as pulmonary fibrosis which is also seen in RA. Both of these conditions are clinically indistinct from methotrexate induced pulmonary fibrosis.

Tutorial

Caplan's syndrome is the occurrence of rheumatoid nodules in the lung in association with pneumoconiosis. Other manifestations include: bronchiolitis obliterans, arytenepiglottitis, tracheitis, pleural fibrosis, phrenic nerve palsy.

Answer 86

D Patients may suffer from hypoglossal nerve palsy.

Wegener's granulomatosis is a large vessel vasculitis that characteristically affects the lung and kidneys. Diagnosis requires the presence of tissue granulomata (caseation is seen in TB). Lung cavitation and renal failure are common. Other presentations include: stuffy nose, collapsed nasal bridge, deafness (conductive due to granuloma in middle ear, or sensorineural due to vasculitis induced neuropathy). Serologically c-ANCA is positive in 80% of people, and p-ANCA in 20–30% of patients. Hypoglossal nerve palsy can result from either compression from skull base granuloma (slightly commoner) or vasculitic ischaemic neuropathy.

Tutorial

Complications include renal failure and pulmonary haemorrhage. Treatment is with high-dose steroids and pulses of cyclophosphamide therapy. Other renal–pulmonary syndromes include SLE and Goodpasture's.

Answer 87

E The standard error of the mean is generally more accurate than the mean.

A normal distribution is a distribution in which all the observations have an equal likelihood of occurring. The mean is the arithmetic average of all the observations, and 2/3 of the observations will lie within 1 SD either side of the mean. The variance is the square of the SD. The SEM is the SD divided by the square root of N, where N is the sample size, and gives a more accurate measure of the standard deviation of the data set.

Tutorial

A normal distribution is one in which all possible values have an equal likelihood of occurring. Consequently, data sets isolating values in a specified range/quartile are a skewed population, to which the majority of simple statistical tests are inapplicable (e.g. arithmetic mean, SD).

Question 88 The following statement is true:

A The sensitivity of a test is determined by the number of true cases identified from the total number of true cases.
B The specificity of a test is the total number of false cases correctly identified from the total number of cases.
C The positive predictive value of a test is the ability of the test to identify correctly the true cases from the total number of true cases.
D A type I error occurs when a null hypothesis is wrongly rejected.
E The value of r, the correlation coefficient, is always >1.

Question 89 The following is true of the odds ratio:

A Is the sum of the relative risk of the event occurring and the relative risk of it not occurring.
B Represents the likely risk of an event occurring being attributable to the specific factor in question.
C If >1 represents a true increased risk.
D Can be confidently interpreted in isolation.
E If negative implies a beneficial effect of the factor of concern.

Question 90 The following is true of a meta-analysis:

A The same trial is analysed in several different ways.
B Gives a more accurate analysis than a single RCT.
C Fundamental trial differences may be obscured in the analysis.
D Should be performed when there are several RCTs on the same subject matter/drug in question.
E Is usually best performed by the investigators of the first RCT on the subject, as they have set the benchmark.

A 45-year-old male with HIV presented with weakness affecting the left upper and lower limbs. On examination he was confused and had a temperature of 38°C (110.4°F). He had recently been treated for a *Pneumocystis carinii* infection. The CD4 count was 150. CT scan of the brain with contrast revealed subcortical atrophy and multiple contrast enhancing ring lesions in the cortex and subcortical areas.

Question 91 The most probable diagnosis is:

A Primary CNS lymphoma.
B Tuberculous meningitis.
C CMV encephalitis.
D Cerebral toxoplasmosis.
E Progressive multifocal leucoencephalopathy.

Answer 88

C The positive predictive value of a test is the ability of the test to identify correctly the true cases from the total number of true cases.

The PPV gives an idea of how good any given test is for correctly identifying all positive cases in the population being investigated.

$$\text{Sensitivity} = \frac{\text{No. of true positives}}{\text{No. of true positives + false negatives}}$$

Tutorial

Type I error = false positive result.
Type II error = false negative assumption.

A negative value for r implies a negative correlation (an inverse relationship).

$$\text{Specificity} = \frac{\text{No. of true negatives}}{\text{No. of true negatives + false positives}}$$

Answer 89

B Represents the likely risk of an event occurring being attributable to the specific factor in question.

The odds ratio is the relative risk of an event occurring due to a specific factor divided by the relative risk of the event not occurring due to the specific factor. The OR can only be interpreted accurately within confidence intervals. An OR of >1 does not support importance of the risk factor in question if the confidence intervals include the value 1. A negative value indicates an inverse relationship.

Tutorial

The OR is way of expressing the increased risk of developing a condition as a result of the particular risk factor.

Answer 90

D Should be performed when there are several RCTs on the same subject matter/drug in question.

Meta-analyses are usually performed when there is a bulk of trial data on a similar subject matter. The meta-analysis is usually performed by an independent party. A proviso is that the trials to be included should all be constructed in a similar way with similar end points. It is not simply an alternative way of looking at the same data sets from one trial. It does not reflect a greater accuracy in the interpretation of the different trial results but gives a consensus view based on the pooling together of all the source data.

Answer 91

D Cerebral toxoplasmosis.

The most probable diagnosis is cerebral toxoplasmosis. The CT scan is consistent with the diagnosis. The subcortical atrophy probably represents HIV encephalopathy (see below). The exact cause of CNS involvement in HIV infection is largely influenced by the CD4 count. Patients with CD4 counts >500 have benign and malignant brain tumours similar to those seen in immunocompetent patients. Patients with a CD4 count of between 200–500 often have cognitive disorders associated with HIV such as HIV dementia and progressive leucoencephalopathy, which are not mass lesions. Patients with a CD4 count <200 have either opportunistic CNS infections or HIV-related cerebral tumours. Opportunistic infections include toxoplasmosis, TB, CMV, and cryptococcal meningitis. Toxoplasmosis is by far the commonest cerebral mass lesion seen in HIV patients and is associated usually with multiple ring enhancing lesions, either in the corticomedullary junction or around the basal ganglia. Patients often have headache, confusion, and fever. Focal neurological signs or seizure are common. The other opportunistic infections rarely result in mass lesions in the absence of disseminated infection.

Tutorial

Primary CNS lymphoma does display some degree of contrast enhancement but it is usually nodular or patchy; however, it may be identical to that seen in toxoplasmosis. Lesions may be multiple and difficult to differentiate from toxoplasmosis. Thallium single photon emission computed tomography (SPECT) has been shown to be useful in differentiating cerebral toxoplasmosis from cerebral lymphoma. Primary CNS lymphoma is rarer than cerebral toxoplasmosis in HIV infection. Generally, patients with multiple ring enhancing lesions on the CT scan with mass effect are treated empirically for *Toxoplasma* infection for 2 weeks with a combination of pyrimethamine and sulphadiazine. Failure of a radiological response (on CT scan) is an indication for brain biopsy to enable an alternative diagnosis such as lymphoma to be made.

A 67-year-old male with dilated cardiomyopathy has breathlessness on walking 50 yards. His medication comprises frusemide 80 mg daily, ramipril 10 mg daily, candesartan 6 mg daily, spironolactone 25 mg daily, bisoprolol 7.5 mg daily and isosorbide mononitrate SR 60 mg daily. On examination the heart rate was 70/min and regular. The blood pressure measured 80/40 mmHg (10.7/5.3 kPa). The JVP was raised. Examination of the precordium revealed a displaced apex in the 6th intercostal space and a forceful right ventricular impulse. Auscultation of the heart revealed a systolic murmur in the mitral area and a third heart sound. On auscultation of the lungs there was evidence of bilateral pleural effusions. The ECG showed LBBB and the left ventricular ejection fraction on the echocardiogram was 25%.

Question 92 The best management step in improving his symptoms is:

A Add digoxin.
B Consider mitral valve repair.
C Increase the dose of bisoprolol.
D Implant a biventricular pacemaker.
E Increase the dose of diuretics.

A 43-year-old male was admitted with a 2-hour history of malaise and nausea. A 12-lead ECG revealed an acute inferior myocardial infarction and third degree AV block. He was an insulin-dependent diabetic. The heart rate at rest was 34/min. The blood pressure was 90/50 mmHg (12/6.7 kPa). Both heart sounds were normal. A temporary pacing wire was inserted via the right superficial femoral vein and the patient was successfully paced.

Question 93 The next management step would be:

A IV heparin.
B IV recombinant tissue plasminogen activator.
C IV metoprolol.
D IV streptokinase.
E IV glyceryl trinitrate.

A 27-year-old journalist returned from a 12-week working period in Kenya with a 2-week history of loss of appetite, fever, and sore throat. On examination she had generalized cervical lymphadenopathy, bright red pharynx without a purulent exudate, and a widespread maculopapular rash. Blood results: Hb 13 g/dl, WCC 7.5×10^9/l, neutrophils 6×10^9/l, lymphocytes 1.3×10^9/l, platelets 180×10^9/l, blood film atypical lymphocytes.

Question 94 The most probable diagnosis is:

A Infectious mononucleosis.
B CMV infection.
C HIV seroconversion.
D Malaria.
E Scarlet fever.

A 50-year-old male presented with central chest pain associated with ST segment depression in the anterior. Troponin T 12 hours after admission was 0.9 ng/l. The patient remained pain free for 3 days and the ECG changes resolved. He was treated with antiplatelet agents, a statin, ACE inhibitor, and a beta-blocker.

Question 95 The most important investigation prior to discharge is:

A Echocardiography.
B Coronary angiography.
C Exercise stress test.
D Measure CRP.
E Myoperfusion scan.

Answer 92

D Implant a biventricular pacemaker.

Biventricular pacemaker is recommended for patients with heart failure who have all of the following:

- NYHA III/IV despite appropriate medical therapy.
- Ejection fraction <25%.
- Co-existing interventricular conduction defect.

Tutorial

Patients with cardiomyopathy and interventricular conduction defects are generally more symptomatic than those with normal conduction due to the resulting desynchronization of ventricular contraction. Pacing both ventricles (RV is paced conventionally; LV is paced via the coronary sinus) helps to resynchronize ventricular contraction and improve functional capacity. Biventricular pacing is only recommended in patients with sinus rhythm (not AF). Biventricular pacing does not alter the prognosis.

Answer 93

B IV recombinant tissue plasminogen activator.

He should be thrombolyzed. In the presence of hypotension, recombinant tissue plasminogen activator is preferred over streptokinase.

Tutorial

See Cardiology section, Questions 9, 10.

Answer 94

C HIV seroconversion.

The diagnosis is between infectious mononucleosis and HIV seroconversion. There are three important factors which favour HIV seroconversion over infectious mononucleosis. Firstly, the patient has a relative lymphopaenia whereas patients with infectious mononucleosis often have lymphocytosis. Secondly, a maculopapular rash is unusual in infectious mononucleosis in the absence of treatment with ampicillin or amoxycillin. Thirdly, whilst sore throat is a feature of both conditions, patients with infectious mononucleosis often have tonsillar exudates which may be absent in HIV seroconversion.

Tutorial

Other features which would normally support HIV seroconversion would be the presence of mucocutaneous ulceration and early onset of diarrhoea (within 3 days of the illness).

Answer 95

B Coronary angiography.

The patient has had a non-ST elevation MI (chest pain and raised troponin in the absence of ST elevation). Such patients have a relatively low risk of in-hospital mortality compared with ST segment elevation MI; however, 6-month mortality exceeds that of patients with ST elevation MI, therefore it is prudent that all appropriate patients with non-ST elevation MI have coronary angiography and revascularization (if required) prior to discharge from hospital. The same applies for patients who present with chest pain and marked ST segment depression even if the troponin is not elevated.

Tutorial

The management in both group of patients is essentially the same and comprises antithrombotic agents (aspirin and clopidogrel), fractionated heparin, and IIB/IIIa platelet receptor blocking agents. In addition, beta-blockers may reduce myocardial oxygen demand. Glyceryl trinitrate infusion is useful in reducing acute ischaemia.

Question 96 A 24-year-old female presented with a 2 cm nodule in the right thyroid lobe associated with cervical lymphadenopathy. She was clinically euthyroid. The next best investigation of choice is:

A Thyroid function tests.
B Fine needle aspiration of the thyroid gland.
C Ultrasound of the thyroid.
D Radioactive thyroid uptake scan.
E CT scan thyroid.

Question 97 A 20-year-old male was admitted with HT, oliguria, and blood and protein in the urine. The serum potassium was 7.4 mmol/l. The immediate management step is:

A Haemodialysis.
B IV actrapid and dextrose 50%.
C Calcium resonium enema.
D IV calcium gluconate.
E Nebulized salbutamol.

A 40-year-old female with dilated cardiomyopathy is seen in the heart failure clinic complaining of a persistent dry cough. Her exercise capacity is 1 mile whilst walking on the flat. She can climb two flights of stairs without difficulty. Her medication consists of ramipril 10 mg daily, aspirin 75 mg daily, carvedilol 6.25 mg twice daily, and frusemide 40 mg daily. On examination the heart rate is 70/min. The blood pressure is 100/60 mmHg (13.3/8 kPa). Both heart sounds are normal and the chest is clear.

Question 98 Her treatment should be altered by:

A Adding spironolactone.
B Substituting ramipril with losartan.
C Reducing carvedilol to 3.125 mg twice daily.
D Doubling the dose of frusemide.
E Adding digoxin.

Question 99 This is a family tree with a very rare condition. The mode of inheritance of this condition is:

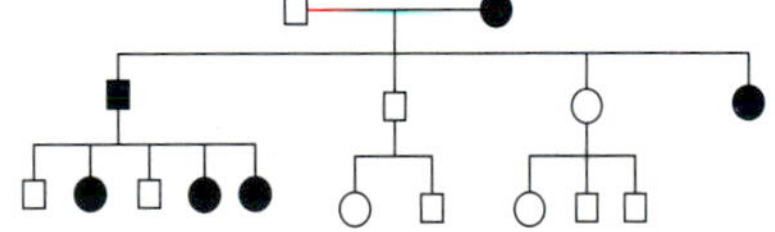

A Autosomal dominant.
B X-linked recessive.
C X-linked dominant.
D Autosomal dominant with incomplete penetrance.
E Autosomal recessive.

A 52-year-old male with noninsulin-dependent diabetes mellitus has a blood pressure of 148/94 mmHg (19.7/12.5 kPa). Fundoscopy reveals evidence of background diabetic retinopathy. The 24 hour urine protein is 1 g. The creatinine is 140 mmol/l.

Question 100 The best treatment in reducing the rate of nephropathy is:

A Losartan.
B Ramipril.
C Insulin.
D Metformin.
E Atenolol.

Answer 96

B Fine needle aspiration of the thyroid gland.

The main aim is to exclude thyroid cancer, which accounts for up to 6.5% of all thyroid lumps. Certain age groups are at particular risk and include those aged <30 years or >60 years. Patients who have had irradiation to the head and neck are also at increased risk. The patient has associated cervical lymphadenopathy, which in this age group raises the suspicion of a papillary cell thyroid carcinoma. Fine needle aspiration is the treatment of choice for making the diagnosis.

Tutorial

Whilst ultrasonography would provide more details about the morphology of the gland, it is not diagnostic. Thyroid scintography is sometimes used by some centres to ascertain the functional status of the gland but in this particular situation it would not provide a diagnosis.

Answer 97

D IV calcium gluconate.

Hyperkalaemia is associated with electrical instability of the heart and may result in ventricular fibrillation or asystole. Urgent management of hyperkalaemia is indicated when the potassium is <7 mmol/l. Urgent treatment is also required at lower serum potassium concentrations if there are ECG changes of hyperkalaemia or evidence of muscle weakness in the context of the raised potassium.The management of hyperkalaemia is tabulated below (*Tutorial*). In urgent cases, the immediate treatment is aimed at preventing cardiac arrest with IV calcium in the form of calcium gluconate or carbonate. The drug acts quickly and its effects last up to 60 min, allowing more definitive measures to control serum potassium levels as shown below, e.g. dextrose and insulin or beta-agonists. In this particular case, the patient has renal failure and the best definitive treatment would be to start haemodialysis.

Tutorial

Management of hyperkalaemia

- Antagonism of membrane actions of potassium:
  - Calcium.
- Drive extracellular potassium into cells:
  - Dextrose and insulin.
  - Sodium bicarbonate if acidotic.
  - Beta-agonists.
- Removal of potassium from cells:
  - Diuretics.
  - Cation exchange resins.
  - Haemodialysis if severe.

Answer 98

B Substituting ramipril with losartan.

The patient is in NYHA functional class II with respect to her symptoms. She is on the correct dose of ramipril and is appropriately being treated with a beta-blocker. The dry cough that the patient is experiencing is almost certainly the side-effect of ramipril. Angiotensin-converting enzyme inhibitors are associated with a dry cough in 15–20% of patients due to increases in circulating bradykinin levels. In such patients the ACE inhibitor should be stopped and substituted with an angiotensin receptor blocker such as losartan.

Tutorial

The efficacy of losartan compared with an ACE inhibitor (captopril) was fully evaluated in the ELITE II study. The study revealed similar mortality rates and similar rates of progression of heart failure when comparing patients on losartan 50 mg daily with those prescribed captopril 50 mg three times daily. The study suggests that losartan is as effective as ACE inhibitors in the management of heart failure. However, the use of losartan in heart failure is still currently reserved for patients who develop side-effects to ACE inhibitors.

Answer 99

C X-linked dominant.

Males and females are affected in all generations, therefore the mode of inheritance could be either autosomal dominant or X-linked dominant. In X-linked states, an affected male passes his X chromosome to all his daughters. His sons only inherit the Y sex chromosome. Therefore, in an X-linked dominant condition the female offspring of an affected male will all inherit the disorder, whereas the males will be free of disease. This is highlighted in the second generation where the first male (affected) has normal sons but all three of his daughters are affected.

Answer 100

A Losartan.

The patient has moderate proteinuria and abnormal renal function. The question specifically relates to the treatment of diabetic nephropathy in a patient with type 2 diabetes mellitus. Whilst ACE inhibitors have been clearly shown to attenuate microalbuminuria in patients without overt nephropathy and to retard progression of nephropathy in those patients with established diabetic nephropathy in type 1 diabetes, the management of nephropathy in type 2 diabetes is still evolving.

Tutorial

It is clear that tight glycaemic control is effective in retarding nephropathy in both type 1 and type 2 diabetes mellitus and that control of hypertension is also necessary in both conditions. In contrast with type 1 diabetes mellitus, there is much less information on the effects of ACE inhibitors in treating diabetic nephropathy in type 2 diabetes mellitus. However, two important studies have shown that in patients with type 2 diabetes, angiotensin receptor blockers are as effective in retarding nephropathy as ACE inhibitors are in type 1 diabetes mellitus. For example, in the RENAAL trial, 1513 patients with type 2 diabetes and nephropathy were randomly assigned to losartan (50 mg titrating up to 100 mg once daily) or placebo, both in addition to conventional antihypertensive therapy (but not ACE inhibitors). Compared to placebo, losartan reduced the incidence of a doubling of the plasma creatinine by 25% and end-stage renal disease by 28%; the mean follow-up was 3.4 years. These benefits were not associated with differences in blood pressure levels between the groups. Subsequent analysis found that the most significant risk factor for progressive kidney disease was the initial degree of proteinuria.

Index

Note: references give the question page number followed by chapter and question numbers in italics (e.g. 181–*14.9*)